MEDICINE, MONOPOLIES, AND MALICE

DR. CHESTER A. WILK

Publisher and Author of 2nd Edition:
Chester A. Wilk, D.C., P.C.
5130 W. Belmont Avenue
Chicago, IL 60641

Library of Congress Cataloging-in-Publication Data

Wilk, Chester A.
    Medicine, monopolies, and malice : how the medical establishment
tried to destroy chiropractic in the U.S. / Chester A. Wilk.
        p. cm.
    Includes bibliographical references and index.
    1. Wilk, Chester A.—Trials, litigation, etc. 2. American Medical
Association—Trials, litigation, etc. 3. Antitrust law—United States.
4. Chiropractic—Law and legislation—United States.

Printed in the United States of America.

10 9 8 7 6 5 4 3 2

CONTENTS

This book is dedicated to my wife, Ardith,
and to my three daughters, Kim, Cathy, and Cindy.
I love them very much and thank them
for their support and sacrifices.
This book is also dedicated to people everywhere,
who deserve honesty and fairness in health care.

ACKNOWLEDGMENTS

I extend deep thanks to Rudy Shur, he is a dear friend, a teacher, and a coach. It was he who saw the human interest story at the core of what had been a simple academic description of events, and insisted that it be brought out to become the heart and soul of the book. He also kept me honest by demanding absolute and complete documentation of virtually every statement I made.

Thank you to Marilyn Beyer and to Amy Tecklenburg for their invaluable editing, which made the manuscript sparkle and come to life.

My heartfelt thanks to attorney George McAndrews and his support team, without whom none of this could have been possible. Thank you also to James W. Bryden, D.C., Patricia B. Arthur, D.C., and Michael D. Pedigo, D.C., my fellow plaintiffs in *Wilk* et al. v. *American Medical Association* et al., and to all the members of the National Chiropractic Antitrust Committee, for their courage and dedication to the cause.

Finally, thank you to my wife, Ardith, for her unwavering love and support.

PREFACE

Chiropractic is a form of health care that respects the body's own natural recuperative capabilities and works to enhance these capabilities through safe, natural means. In the 100 years of its formal existence as a profession, chiropractic has proved itself to be safer, more cost-effective, and, most important of all, therapeutically superior to other types of treatment for problems of the musculoskeletal system. Government-sponsored studies from countries around the world—including the United States—attest to its clinical superiority. Its colleges have been found by leading medical educators to offer superior facilities and training. And surveys have found that chiropractic patients are three times more likely to be satisfied with their care than patients of medical doctors are.

If chiropractic has all these advantages, why doesn't everyone know it? Why are medical doctors more likely to refer patients with back pain to orthopedists and neurologists, rather than to chiropractors? And why is it that most American hospitals not only have no chiropractic departments, but do not have even a single affiliated chiropractor—in spite of the overwhelming evidence of chiropractic's superiority?

These were some of the questions I asked myself over the past forty years, as I watched my profession struggle and grow, and as I myself struggled and grew within it. When I finally learned the answers, it changed my life. I learned that all of the misconceptions, broken promises, and slammed doors we chiropractors found ourselves facing every day were no accident, but a product of a calculated campaign by organized medicine that meant to do no less than to destroy our profession.

This book is the story of my journey to find the truth. It is a

story of conspiracy and intrigue I once would have thought
existed only in the pages of detective novels—certainly not in
the everyday world I live in. It is also the story of the legal drama
that consumed fourteen years of my life, and of the many ex-
traordinary individuals I came to know, admire, and value as a
result. Finally, it is the story of what I believe to be one of the
most important and fiercely fought battles in the history of
health care in the United States.

                                                    Chester A. Wilk

1

BEFORE THE STORM

I t was a typical winter day in Chicago, December 9, 1980. The air was cool, with a steady breeze coming in from the east, and the sky was overcast. At the Cumberland Avenue station, I parked the car, and the two of us ascended the stairway to board the elevated train that would take us into the heart of the city. The ride was a familiar one that I had taken dozens of times in my life. But on this particular day it felt strikingly different. I breathed deeply, partly to etch the moment into my memory, but more to settle the excitement I felt in the pit of my stomach.

My wife was with me. She had come both to share this experience and to provide moral support, as she had so often done through the difficult years that had preceded this day. Ardith and I sat silently, holding hands, as the elevated train headed southeast toward the Loop. We gazed vacantly as we passed high above the city, engrossed in our thoughts. As the elevated train reached Ashland Avenue, it descended into a tunnel and became a subway. Thirty-five minutes later, we got off the train at the Dearborn Avenue station.

We took the escalator, which went up only part of the way, and then we climbed the stairs to the street. As we walked side by side, I felt my wife's hand trembling in mine, partly from the coolness of the breeze coming in across Lake Michigan, but also from her nervousness and apprehension.

Directly in front of us was the Everett McKinley Dirksen Building, Chicago's federal building. This imposing edifice is one of the most modern architectural structures in the city, with large windows and a lot of glass on the street level. The building stands tall and stately, befitting the courts and offices it houses. Inside, on the ground level, is a spacious open area, with ceilings about three stories high. We found an elevator that carried us to the twenty-first floor.

To the right, down the hallway from the elevator and next to the heavy walnut door of room 2119, a brushed-aluminum plate with deeply etched Gothic-style lettering identified the domain of the Honorable Judge Nicholas J. Bua. We stepped inside the empty courtroom. It was nine o'clock in the morning, exactly one hour before the federal district court session was scheduled to begin, and we were the first to arrive. My eyes connected for a moment with my wife's. Nothing was spoken by either of us; we were both deep in our own thoughts. Still hand in hand, we seated ourselves in the next-to-last row on the right. We had sixty minutes to wait, and to think.

The courtroom was impressive—simple, classic, and magnificently appointed. The walls were richly paneled in walnut, and the floor was covered with eye-pleasing neutral carpeting. It was a place devoid of windows, by design completely removed from the bustling streets of the city. The judge's bench was the room's most prominent feature. It was well lighted and built on a raised platform to overlook the courtroom, and it appeared very imposing even when it was empty. Clearly, this was where the most important activities of the court took place. On the right side of the room, in the center and on a slightly elevated platform, was the box for seating twelve chosen jury members. On the main floor, directly in front of and perpendicular to the judge's bench, was a long walnut table flanked by chairs intended to accommodate the various legal counsel expected for this trial. The rest of the courtroom was furnished with dark walnut benches for the audience. These could comfortably seat about 100 people.

Ardith seemed preoccupied, uneasy, but if in any way she questioned the developments that had brought us to this point, she did not mention it. I sensed worry and stress behind the expression on her face. We were poised on the threshold of a great courtroom drama, and she dreaded the possibility of failure. She knew, better than anyone else, the cause that had been growing within me for the past seven years, and that now consumed me. This was a battle that had to be fought and won at all costs. Ardith knew what a crushing personal defeat it would be for me if we were to fail in this, and at times it was an effort for her to subdue the uncomfortable fear that threatened her composure—fear for me and my security, both personal and professional, and fear for our well-being and that of our three young daughters. The small hand I held, cold yet sweaty, still trembled at times. Her other hand clutched the handle of her handbag, just as firmly as she clung to the belief that we were doing the right thing. Her conviction had been fueled and strengthened by the fervent prayers she had raised over the years for divine guidance, for the strength to see this through, and for direction to people who could bring this matter to justice, and her strong faith upheld her now. And so, with much determination, she fixed her mind on courage and ultimate victory. This wonderful woman believed in me, and that was my greatest strength of all. In her heart she knew beyond every doubt that it was right for us to be in this place.

As did I. Nothing is more empowering than knowing you are right, and I had not the slightest doubt that our cause was right and that we were championing the truth. This had already motivated me for several years, and I knew it was the one thing that would sustain me for as long as necessary. After seven years of anticipation and preparation, we nervously yet eagerly awaited the beginning of a trial that was destined to have a major impact on our lives and on the course of an entire profession. These moments of silence before the trial gave me time to pause for reflection, and in those moments, the sequence of events that had led to this point passed through my mind. Where had the time gone? I wondered. And yet it felt as if I had been waiting for an eternity.

We were here to take on the greatest powers in the American medical establishment. I knew that if we won, it could revolutionize health care; if we lost, I could lose everything, professionally and personally. There was no question this would be the greatest fight of my life. Who would ever have thought that this would be my destiny? I had always been somewhat shy and unassuming, not aggressive and not assertive, certainly an unlikely candidate for initiating a court action such as this. Why me? I had always considered myself a very average, ordinary person. There were many others who were more articulate and knowledgeable. Yet here I was. Somehow fate had thrown me into the middle of what I believed to be one of the most important health-related legal actions in American history. It has been said that there are not that many unusual people in the world, but only ordinary people who have unusual opportunities and embrace them. I guess that is what happened to me.

* * *

In 1949, when I was nineteen years old, I was in my third semester of study at the Chicago College of Optometry. In those days, no aptitude tests or even career counseling was available to help young adults determine the kind of work for which they might be best suited.

My parents had always worked very hard, up to sixteen hours a day. My dad worked as a painter and wallpaper-hanger, and together my parents owned and operated a small mom-and-pop grocery store that was part of the Midwest Grocery chain. The store was located on Cicero Avenue, on the northwest side of Chicago, and our family lived in an apartment at the back of the store. This was not the modern type of grocery store equipped with wide aisles and shopping carts. In those days, customers would come in and tell the grocer what they wanted, and the grocer would collect it for them, in the meantime exchanging friendly conversation until the bill was tallied and the transaction completed. Often, patrons who chanced to meet inside gathered near the front window to chat. As a youth, I had my own job to do in this family-operated business; I stocked the shelves with the nonperishable goods, and I also had the job of saturating the neighborhood with weekly circulars that advertised the sale prices on goods received from the central wholesaler. I saw how hard my parents worked to make a meager living, and I felt I had to do better. My plan was to get a professional education, not to spend years in college only to end up with a job a high school graduate could have. My American Dream also included autonomy; I did not want to spend years in a job working toward retirement only to someday have my fate in the hands of someone younger than I, who might decide I wasn't needed anymore.

We purchased our perishable grocery items from independent merchants. One of them was a peddler named Sam Catoni, who used to deliver fresh fruit and vegetables to my parents' store. I never asked Mr. Catoni for career advice, but he volunteered it anyway. In fact, he went further than that; he actually pushed what he believed to be the ideal profession—optometry—as something he said I could make a good living doing.

"You don'a get your hands'a dirty; you keepa you' hands'a clean," he said, in his heavily accented English. "You don'a see blood. You don'a cut anyone open. You fix'a the lenses. You sit by a machine'a an'a put the lenses in'a front of the eye; an' you'a fit lenses. A nice clean job. An optometrist—that'sa what you should be!"

I had no idea if I would like optometry, but Mr. Catoni's suggestion sounded good and made an impact on me. So on the basis of his advice, and with the approval of my family, I took the plunge and decided to pursue optometry.

I found the studies to be a grind. Subconsciously, I knew something was missing for me, but I could not put my finger on what it was. I tried to look at my college studies as an interim period leading to a better time, imagining that I would care more for optometry as a profession when I could finally take my position in the workplace.

In a serious effort to achieve academically, I often studied late into the night. As a result, I developed many stress-related back pains. Most of the pain was between my shoulders. It was a burning pain that would not let up for days at a time.

The pains in my back became severe enough that I went to our family medical doctor seeking relief. He advised me to press on the sore muscles with my thumbs to release the tension. That didn't help, so I went to another doctor. The second physician wrote me a prescription for a painkiller.

I took this prescription to a local pharmacist by the name of Walter Kopec. He had a nice, modern drugstore located on the northwest side of Chicago, on Fullerton Avenue just east of Laramie. Mr. Kopec was a sweet and gentle man in his late forties, small of stature. Because of a short right leg, he walked slowly, with a limp. Mr. Kopec was well respected in the neighborhood and had a loyal clientele. The local people trusted him so much that they often consulted with him before visiting their medical doctors. On this day, he looked at my handwritten prescription rather intently for a few moments, then looked at me, then back at the prescription in his hand. After a thoughtful moment, he asked, "Is this for you?"

"Yes, it is," I replied.

He read the prescription once again, then said, "This is a very strong painkiller. If you take this kind of medication now, at your age, what will become of you when you're forty?" He shrugged his shoulders, shook his head as if to say no, and said, "Well, I can fill this prescription for you. It's up to you."

This took me completely by surprise. I was struck by the man's unusual expression of compassion and concern for me, which apparently took precedence over the sale of his merchandise.

"Since you put it that way, I won't need to take it," I replied. Then I thanked him for his concern and his honesty, adding that he might have lost a sale, but he had gained one person's trust and respect. I have never forgotten the depth of his concern. I could not have guessed then that this experience would change the direction of my life.

At home, I told my mother what Mr. Kopec had said when he saw my prescription. And then she said, "Listen. The first doctor said you should press on the sore spots in your back with your thumbs. Why don't you go see Dr. Nowak? He is an expert with back pain. Let him press on them for you, since that's the kind of thing he does for a living."

Dr. John Nowak was a chiropractor. He was a very distinguished looking man in his fifties. He was always well dressed and he sported a mustache, which somehow added to his professional image. Whenever he entered a room, he attracted attention. He had a strong presence.

I didn't know why I hadn't thought of it. Until that moment, the subject of chiropractic had never come up as a possible treatment for my back pains. I thought my mother's suggestion was a good idea.

I made an appointment with Dr. Nowak, and a couple of days later I went to his office for my first chiropractic adjustment. The examination began with a routine patient history, which the doctor took himself. After that, he ushered me into the treatment room, where he asked me more specific questions. Then he instructed me to strip to the waist, lie against a hydraulic table, and relax. The padded table was lowered into a horizontal position, with me prone upon it. The doctor ran his fingers and palms along my spine, feeling with hands of experience both the vertebrae and the muscles. Then, with a quick, deft thrust of his hands, he gave me my first chiropractic adjustment. With the movement, I heard a popping sound, but it was not even slightly uncomfortable for me.

Dr. Nowak worked on my entire spine. Then he raised the hydraulic table and instructed me to lie on my back on a different table. While I was in that supine position, he adjusted my neck. Finally, he had me lie on my side as he took my leg forward, contracted my hip, and adjusted my lower back. He did this first on one side and then on the other.

It was quite an experience. I will never forget how I went to the doctor's office with a pain in my back that I had been experiencing for weeks, and walked out feeling better and immeasurably relieved. After only a couple of these treatments, the pain I had suffered for the past year completely disappeared. I was very impressed that Dr. Nowak could accomplish so quickly what two medical doctors had not been able to accomplish at all. And we talked about it.

Dr. Nowak explained to me that a chiropractic adjustment is a specific type of manual manipulation of the spinal vertebrae for the purpose of removing what are called *vertebral subluxations*. An adjustment makes the spine more movable, improves nerve activity, and allows the body to utilize its own natural healing power. During an adjustment, a patient will often hear (as I did) clicking sounds from within the spine in the adjusted area. Dr. Nowak told me that many patients welcome these sounds because they recognize them as part of the healing process, since some relief from pain is often immediate.

Possibly because I was so enthusiastic over having my pain relieved, Dr. Nowak suggested that I give some thought to changing professional directions and becoming a chiropractor. He urged me to visit the nearby National College of Chiropractic. Initially, his advice made no impression on me at all. I listened to him casually and dismissed the idea without even considering it. After all, I was already in the middle of my third semester at the Chicago College of Optometry. I was in a four-year program there, and after the current semester I would have only five semesters left before I was to become a licensed optometrist. At this point in my life, such a change in direction seemed unrealistic.

During a subsequent visit to Dr. Nowak's office, he asked me if I had gone to look over the chiropractic college as he had suggested. I admitted I had not. This time, he was more adamant, and he insisted that I should not disregard the suggestion without giving it the slightest consideration.

"Don't be so stubborn!" he said. "Listen to me. The chiropractic college is just down the street—before closing your mind, go there and see for yourself. What have you got to lose? How can you know how you feel about it if you don't give the idea a chance?"

More to get Dr. Nowak off my back than because I had any real interest in becoming a chiropractor, I stopped by the college for a visit. The National College of Chiropractic was housed in an old five-story structure located only one mile south of Dr. Nowak's office, on the southwest corner of Ashland Avenue and Warren Boulevard. The entire college at that time was contained within that building and its basement. Although I had no appointment, when I told the person at the reception desk that I was considering studying chiropractic and had come to see the college, I was welcomed and warmly greeted by the college president himself. He was Dr. Joseph Janse, affectionately called J.J., a man who I later learned was something of a legend in the profession. He graciously conducted me on a tour of the college, and I was very impressed both with the facilities and with the profound sincerity and dedication of this man. Dr. Janse radiated charisma. His enthusiasm and genuine affection for his profession were contagious. There was no question that he derived great satisfaction from his work, that chiropractic was a labor of love for him.

* * *

I learned much about chiropractic that day, and gained a better understanding of my experience with Dr. Nowak's treatments. I learned that the spine is a biomechanical structure, which means that it is part of a living and vibrant machine—the body— and that it is involved in moving, pulling, pushing, flexing, and extending in different directions, as we walk, run, climb, bend, lift, twist, stoop, squat, reach, pull, and push. (*See* Good Structure Equals Good Function on page 10.) The vertebrae, the bones of the spine, slide within a normal range of motion, and thus act as joints. Discs between the vertebrae serve as shock absorbers. The nerves and blood vessels exiting from the spine are also involved in the biomechanical function of the body, and they help in the body's ability to move muscles and joints, and also in organ function. All the different parts of the spine are naturally subjected to injury, stress, fatigue, and so on, which may affect the vertebral joints' ability to function normally. If that happens, local congestion, swelling, restricted motion, muscle spasm, and pain may follow, impairing the biomechanics of the spine. This in turn restricts joint motion and causes nerve irritation and more discomfort. This is what chiropractors refer to as a *vertebral subluxation complex.* Subluxations of vertebrae can occur anywhere in the spine, and can range from minor to severe. However, even a slight misalignment that does not directly affect the spinal cord may create disturbances in the nerves of the spine, and through them, elsewhere in the body. A chiropractor may adjust the vertebrae in an effort to remove such nerve disturbances, thereby permitting the body to function in a better state of health.

If a vertebral subluxation is in the upper part of the neck, neck pain and headaches are likely; if it is in the lower neck, it may irritate the nerves that extend into the arms; if it is between the shoulder blades, it may cause pain to radiate between the ribs to the front; and if it is in the lower back, pain may extend down the legs. The level of the subluxation affects the location of the problem. Nerves involved in a subluxation not only cause pain, but may also affect the health and integrity of different organs, including the heart, stomach, and lungs, which get their nerve supply from the involved nerves. Such structural problems may be less receptive to medications and more receptive to structurally related treatments, and there is no finer and safer approach than skillful chiropractic adjustments.

A chiropractic adjustment is a specific type of high-velocity manual manipulation of the spinal vertebrae for the purpose of removing subluxations. The spine has a normal range of motion, and an adjustment consists of a precise, swift movement of a vertebra or vertebrae into the paraphysiological range of movement—the outer limits of the spine's normal range of motion.

Good Structure
Equals Good Function

The laws of physics tell us that if you alter the structure of an object, you may alter its ability to perform certain of its designated functions. Similarly, if the structure of the body is altered, its functioning may be affected—especially if the alteration affects the spine, from which nerves extend to all of the various structures of the body.

Dogs, cats, and other animals seem to know this instinctively. They naturally stretch their own bodies, as if they know that correct or improved body structure will improve their bodies' health and functioning. Laboratory experiments show that by flexing or extending their spines, dogs and cats can slow down or speed up, respectively, the flow of blood to the different organs in the body. Hence, "rolling up" can cause a cat to relax and fall asleep, while standing up and stretching can have an awakening effect. This illustrates the influence of the spine on the nervous system for one's overall health and well-being.

Doctors of chiropractic employ a method of healing that pays particular attention to the structural and neurological aspects of the body, particularly the spine, in the prevention and treatment of human ailments. One premise of chiropractic is that good body structure and spinal mechanics, good nerve function, and regular chiropractic adjustments play a significant role in assisting the body to function better and have greater resistance to physical breakdown and disease.

This stretches the ligaments that hold the vertebrae together. It is the elastic resistance of the ligaments that causes the adjustment to take place, making the spine more movable and improving nerve activity, which in turn enhances the body's natural ability to heal itself. The doctor of chiropractic requires a great deal of practice in spinal adjusting to acquire the skill and competence necessary. For this reason, the adjustments should be done only by full-time chiropractic practitioners who have had years of specialized training and who also continually refresh and upgrade their education and skills in this area.

A Doctor of Chiropractic (D.C.) may use his or her own judgment, in keeping with the regulations various states may impose, to use other approaches in tandem with the chiropractic spinal adjustment. He or she may prescribe corrective exercises, physical therapy, dietary regulation, nutritional supplementation, or restriction of activity, or advise rest or even improvements in hygienic care. In fact, chiropractors may utilize any therapeutic measures except drugs or surgery. While state laws vary in regard to what chiropractors may employ in therapy, the chiropractic adjustment, which is the primary mode of treatment, is recognized in all states where chiropractic is licensed.

Chiropractic is wellness-oriented. That is, it strives to maximize the body's own natural and inherent healing power; symptoms are eliminated by treating the patient's underlying problem. This is in contrast to the "crisis-care" approach of current medicine, which too often treats ailments by seeking to eliminate symptoms, and ignores underlying causes. When only the symptoms are treated, the underlying problem may never be fully corrected, and over the long term, the symptoms may tend to return. (*See* The Right Cure for the Illness on page 12.) Critics of this approach to medicine therefore view it as "sickness care" rather than health care. Many studies show that chiropractic provides more lasting and permanent results for certain health care problems than conventional medicine. This is because chiropractic works to improve the body's overall health; the better a person's underlying health, the stronger the body's natural healing ability is, and the less likely the body is to break down or to succumb to illness.

In the same vein, chiropractors have historically opposed the indiscriminate and dangerous use of pharmaceuticals and the institution of mandated, rather than individually or objectively evaluated, immunization programs. Even prior to the incident in Mr. Kopec's drugstore, I had been sensitive to the overmedication of our society and the dangers of mandatory immunization programs. In fact, I had a sister whom I never knew because she died as a result of complications following a diphtheria vaccination.

In 1926, my parents lived in Detroit. My sister Elsie, then three

The Right Cure for the Illness

There are four major types of health care treatments that are commonly used to restore and maintain health; these are surgical (surgery), pharmaceutical (medications), psychological (counseling), and biomechanical (therapeutic body manipulations). Proper health care demands that all four of these be honestly and objectively evaluated, and considered on the basis of their respective merits, for a particular ailment. Then the most conservative treatment that is consistent with safety and effectiveness should be used.

The overutilization of drugs and surgery, with the consequent numbers of drug reactions, extended hospital stays, and complications from unnecessary surgery, point to the need for a more conservative overall approach to health care. In short, drugs and surgery should be resorted to only when natural and drug-free methods cannot do at least as well.

To determine the most appropriate treatment for a particular problem, certain important issues must be addressed. The treatment of choice ought to be the one that is the most therapeutically effective, safe, and cost-efficient. The key to choosing successful treatment is to be properly informed. Briefly, one must consider:

- *What is the most conservative care that is appropriate?*
- *Can the care be accomplished without drugs and surgery?*
- *Is the care effective?*
- *Have all available health care disciplines been totally considered?*

Most experts agree that if an ailment is psychologically based, it is likely to be responsive to psychological treatment; an ailment requiring surgical intervention is generally best treated surgically; an ailment requiring pharmacological treatment is most successfully treated with drugs; and a structurally related ailment will probably respond best to structural or biomechanical treatments. People who are aware of these general principles

> *already have the understanding they need to utilize health care options more intelligently.*
>
> *Suppose a patient had cancer somewhere in his body. Would psychological counseling remove it? Would taking medications correct it? Would getting spinal adjustments correct it? Most of us would probably agree that early detection and a combination of surgical removal and medical treatment of the cancer is the best known treatment. Thus, surgery and medical chemotherapy would be the treatments of choice for most patients with cancer.*
>
> *Now consider the patient whose problem is of a structural nature, the symptoms of which may include rigid and painful muscles and joints, and irritated nerves in the area. Would bombarding his body with drugs correct the problem? Or would it merely mask the symptoms—and perhaps even create the potential for other complications or drug dependence? Would surgery be the answer? It follows that the logical choice for many structurally related ailments is a treatment that will correct the underlying structural problem. This is the realm of most chiropractic care.*

years old, was recovering from diphtheria. In that condition, she should never have been given a vaccination, but my mother went along with what the family doctor advocated. The M.D. administered a diphtheria shot in spite of the little girl's weakened condition. Elsie died the next day in my mother's arms.

A year later, my sister Lottie died at the age of eleven, of scarlet fever—again, ironically, following a doctor's intervention. A doctor was trying to coerce her into eating her food, and told her that if she didn't eat, he would put her in the hospital. Lottie said "Ouch!" and collapsed; within two minutes she was dead. My mother and my older sister Angeline, who were there at the time, believed the fear of going to the hospital upset Lottie so much that she died.

Interestingly, I would never have been born but for the deaths of my sisters. Having lost two children, my mother decided to have one more, and three years later, in 1930, I was born. Because of the tragic story of Elsie's unnecessary death, I came to share the view of many chiropractors who are opposed to mandatory immunization programs. While I am not absolutely opposed to shots, I believe that in some situations, they can cause more problems than they are worth, and their use should meet a stringent cost/benefit/risk analysis.

*   *   *

As my tour of the chiropractic college went on, I loved everything I saw and heard, and my eyes were opened to the realization that optometry was not at all what I was looking for. In fact, it seemed almost as though I could hear the very walls of the chiropractic college calling to me, in a very special way, to enroll. I had never before experienced such a conviction or a feeling toward a teaching institution. I had walked into the college with little thought of becoming a chiropractor. When I walked out that afternoon, I was totally convinced that I could do nothing else.

Returning home that afternoon, I announced my decision to my parents and told them I was quitting optometry immediately. They must have been somewhat stunned by this sudden announcement, but they took it in stride and supported my change of heart. Of course, they loved me, and they accepted my decision with the philosophy that it was I who would have to live with whatever I chose as a profession, so it had better be something I would be happy doing. Most people work to live. If I could live to work, loving what I was doing, my life would be enriched, satisfying, and all the more fulfilling.

My sister, on the other hand, was not at all receptive to my choice. Angeline is fifteen years older than I am. She was married and had a home of her own by this time. But I was still her baby brother, and she felt a need to look out for me. She did everything she could to talk me out of this decision and to convince me to remain enrolled in optometry school.

"You don't want to go to a chiropractic college," Ange said— although she offered no reason why, other than that she considered optometry to be a more prestigious profession. She felt I was lowering myself somehow by choosing chiropractic.

"I was proud of you going to optometry, but I don't think much of chiropractic," she told me. "Don't quit. Stay!" At that time, she did not believe in chiropractic.

There were to be no more doubts on my part, however; I would not be dissuaded. My thoughts took a 180-degree turn the day I decided to become a chiropractor, and I have never regretted it for a moment. It took some time—in fact years—but eventually, my sister also supported my choice and even became a chiropractic patient and an enthusiastic supporter of chiropractic.

The College of Optometry was predictably less pleased by my decision to quit. The college catalog clearly stated that if I withdrew prior to midterm exams, I was entitled to a refund of half the semester's tuition. At first, however, the administration balked at refunding the money. They even tried to hustle me into becoming both an optometrist and a chiropractor. But I had no interest in becoming a jack-of-all-trades. Eventually, I successfully recovered half of the semester's tuition, and I walked away without once looking back. Then I took a temporary job for four weeks as I waited for the new semester to begin at the National College of Chiropractic.

*   *   *

In 1949, the year I enrolled, the chiropractic curriculum required four and a half years to complete. It was a sophisticated, comprehensive program covering anatomy, physiology, chemistry, pathology, bacteriology, public health, dermatology, neurology, pediatrics, radiology, diagnosis, and symptomatology. The anatomy courses were divided into various specialties. And, of course, chiropractic techniques and principles were taught exhaustively. Since chiropractors do not use drugs or surgery, pharmacological and surgical courses were not included in the curriculum. But study of the toxicology of drugs was included, to enable doctors of chiropractic to recognize drug reactions in the patients they treated. There was also clear and emphatic consideration given to the kinds of afflictions that needed to be referred to medical doctors. A course in jurisprudence, which taught ethical principles and legal issues, was also required. The training, I felt, was outstanding and comprehensive, and it would compare favorably even today with that offered at the finest medical schools. (See Chiropractic Education on page 16.)

I was surprised to discover that the most common incentive for students to enroll in chiropractic colleges was a personal experience of success with chiropractic treatment after the failure

Chiropractic Education

The Doctor of Chiropractic degree today requires two years of preprofessional college education, followed by four academic years of resident study consisting of more than 4,200 hours in the classroom. During the first two years, chiropractic programs concentrate on study of the basic sciences, just as medical programs do. But while the second half of the program for medical doctors focuses extensively on drugs and surgery, the third and fourth years of chiropractic programs concentrate on spinal analysis, spinal manipulation, orthopedics, physical therapy, radiology, neurology, and nutrition.

Chiropractic colleges devote much of their curricula to the study of the neuromusculoskeletal system of human beings, which consists of nerves, muscles, bones, and joints, including the spine. It deserves this attention, because the musculoskeletal system makes up 60 percent of the human body's systems in terms of body mass. The extensive training, understanding, and qualification chiropractors receive in this area account for their great success in treating neuromusculoskeletal disorders, without exposing patients to the hazards of drugs and surgery. This is why chiropractic is the best and safest approach to the treatment of many cases of muscle and joint pain, loss of normal joint dynamics (movement), and related conditions.

of orthodox medical care. This could only be attributed to the fact that there are many health problems that are structural in nature and that see minimal improvement, at best, when treated medically. Although spinal manipulation is an ancient art, chiropractic was still something of a new field in 1949, a system of therapy formally founded as recently as 1895. It was not yet widely known, understood, or accepted. Chiropractic colleges had to vigorously pursue the recruitment of students, and admission requirements were therefore not as stringent as they are today.

The past fifty years have seen an explosion of knowledge and technology in nearly every field. The world has been quick to grasp changes in technology. But the acceptance of new knowledge is something that takes place much more slowly. For example, there was a time when 16 percent of women who gave birth died from a disease known as *puerperal sepsis,* or childbed fever. Today, we know that those deaths were the result of infections caused by bacteria that were introduced by the unclean hands of physicians. Dr. Ignaz Semmelweiss (1818–1865) discovered that simply by washing his hands, he could reduce the mortality rate of his maternity patients to only 1 percent, the lowest death rate there had ever been in the hospital in which he worked. He tried to proclaim this discovery to the world, but was contemptuously regarded as a quack by his colleagues, and his teaching was blindly rejected. When he published the book *The Etiology, the Concept, and the Prophylaxis of Childbed Fever,* which provided overwhelming proof of his doctrine, he provoked even greater hostility from his medical contemporaries. Not until several years after Semmelweiss's death did the medical community become convinced of the validity of his discovery, and all doctors began routinely washing their hands.[1] In spite of overwhelming evidence, physicians were reluctant to accept a simple and obvious truth, and no one knows how many patients died or were harmed as a result. It was not particularly surprising, then, that the chiropractic approach to health care took many years to gain popular acceptance.

* * *

I had no sooner finished college and completed the Illinois state board licensing examination than I was drafted into the Army for a two-year stint, beginning in February 1953. A student deferment from military service had afforded me the time necessary to complete my education, but the Korean conflict was the political crisis of the day, and every eligible young man was being drafted. At that time, chiropractors (unlike medical doctors and registered nurses) did not qualify to be commissioned as officers, so I was sent to Camp Roberts in California, where I was trained and assigned to the infantry branch as a private. Later, I managed to get myself transferred into the medical corps as a corpsman. When Camp Roberts was closed, seven months after I arrived, I was transferred to Fort Lewis in Washington.

At Fort Lewis, I was initially assigned to a field medical company. Later, quite by accident, I got transferred to the 16th Signal Corps, and I awaited the processing of orders that would send me to Fort Sam Houston, in Texas, to attend radio school. By the time I was to finish that military occupational training, there would be less than six months remaining before my scheduled discharge. It seemed ludicrous to me that I should be slotted into that kind of occupational specialty in the signal corps. I had no background, interest, or propensity for such an assignment. There is an old saying that there are three ways to do things: the right way, the wrong way, and the Army way. I was not the first person who questioned the wisdom of the Army way!

I spoke with and subsequently received a letter from Colonel John Yuckman, M.D., the commanding officer of the main post dispensary. Colonel Yuckman supported chiropractic, and his letter indicated that my services could be used in the physical therapy unit. With that letter in hand, I went to the regimental post headquarters and spoke with a corporal, explaining to him that I was a chiropractor, licensed in the state of Illinois, and capable of serving my country in a far more useful capacity in the medical corps than in a signal unit. He agreed that my request had a sound basis and submitted my name for a transfer.

Working in the physical therapy unit at the post dispensary, I had my first opportunity since college graduation to function in a capacity where I had some degree of expertise. This is not to imply that I was given the freedom to practice chiropractic there; chiropractic had not been validated by the military powers that be as appropriate treatment. The unit was strictly confined to physical therapy techniques; chiropractic manipulations were not utilized. Since the dispensary had no use for chiropractic therapy, and since I did not want to face any repercussions from doing something officially considered unacceptable, I chose not to reveal to any of the servicemen who came into the dispensary that I was licensed in chiropractic. And so the time passed and I served my military obligation unremarkably—until one day only three months before my scheduled date of discharge.

A master sergeant suffering from neck and upper back pain had been receiving daily treatments in our physical therapy unit for over a month. His discomfort was so severe that it was causing him to lose sleep, and it was really getting him down psychologically. Physiotherapy, massage, shortwave diathermy (deep-heat treatment), and ultrasonic therapy—all standard medical therapies—were used in treatment, but nothing helped his condition or even slightly reduced his pain. Instead, the pain was getting worse. As time progressed, the sergeant could no longer sleep at night except in short naps, and as his pain persisted, his frustration increased, until finally he was quite beside himself with desperation. Somewhere, and I will never know where, he learned what my real profession was.

"Are you a chiropractor?" he asked me one morning.

"Yes, I am," I replied.

He looked earnestly at me. "Then why don't you give me a chiropractic treatment? The pain is intolerable. I can't take it anymore—I've got to have something done." He was pleading. My anguish in that moment was profound. I knew I had both the training and the ability to help a man who was in acute distress, yet I was prevented by bureaucratic regulations from using the opportunity. I strongly believed that American servicemen were not being treated fairly, because men such as this, who so clearly needed chiropractic care, were denied it. This did not make sense to me, nor did it to the sergeant.

"I wish I could," I explained, trying to keep the emotion out of my voice, "but understand that chiropractic is not recognized here, and getting any medical doctor to officially recommend it here would be unlikely. It is against the medical policy of the Army." I shook my head with regret. "I'm truly sorry, but I just can't do it unless you can get a medical consultation slip signed by a medical doctor. I would have to have the authorization in writing."

The sergeant rubbed his chin. "Suppose I get a consultation slip signed by a medical doctor. Then would you give me your chiropractic treatment?"

"Indeed I would!"

The sergeant always had one of the earliest appointments in the day. I do not know how he accomplished it, but the next morning he produced written authorization requesting a course of spinal adjustments, and the order was signed by an M.D. I was amazed and pleasantly surprised.

That morning the sergeant received his first adjustment. This may well have been the first chiropractic adjustment ever done in the medical facility of this Army post. The physical therapy tables available in the dispensary worked fine for this treatment. I adjusted his upper spine, and his vertebrae popped loudly. He remarked that he felt instantly improved, but we had yet to see what the long-term results would be.

The following day, the sergeant did not show up for his usual morning appointment. He hadn't missed being there, and on time, for over a month. As the morning went on, I became uneasy and increasingly concerned, though I tried not to show it. I found myself glancing frequently at a clock on the wall as I went about the morning routine.

The minutes stretched into hours. Suddenly, at noon—more than two hours after the sergeant's scheduled appointment—the door was thrown open and he came striding briskly in, beaming from ear to ear. He had overslept, and it was the first good night's sleep he had had in over a month. He was so overjoyed and so deeply grateful that he had tears in his eyes. His pain was almost gone. After only two more treatments over the following days, he was completely free of pain.

The sergeant became a virtual one-man public relations machine for chiropractic on that Army post, and in his position he came into contact with a great number of people. The news spread like a wildfire! In a short time, some of the highest ranking brass on the post were coming in with similar pains and requesting adjustments of the spine. In each case, I demanded—and received—a written consultation slip authorizing spinal manipulative adjustments. It occurred to me that questions could potentially be raised by higher-up medical brass as to my practice of chiropractic in this Army facility. I even feared it might anger some of them enough to have me transferred out of the dispensary. But that never happened. Having every request authorized and signed by an M.D. gave me justification in case I needed it, but no questions of any kind ever surfaced. Whether that was because of the high-ranking individuals I was treating or because some of the medical doctors, like the dispensary's commanding officer, Colonel Yuckman, supported the practice of chiropractic, I will never know.

It happened that the master sergeant I had treated first was assigned in the department that handled discharges on Fort

Lewis. As a gesture of appreciation for the help I had given him, he told me that when the time came for my discharge, he would expedite paperwork for me and give my out-processing top priority. He was true to his word, and I did not have to stand in line. It was a happy day for me when I accepted my honorable discharge and hurried back home to Chicago.

* * *

It was 1955, and it was springtime. With my military obligation behind me, I felt both confident and eager to get started in my chiropractic practice. I had found a location for my new office on Belmont Avenue, just off Long Avenue, in the vicinity of the neighborhood where I grew up.

One day I stopped by the neighborhood drugstore to visit my old pharmacist, Mr. Kopec.

"Good morning Mr. Kopec. Do you remember me?"

He looked at me and said, "Yes, I believe I do. I see a lot of people, and you look familiar."

"You have a good memory. Chet Wilk is my name. I've been gone—I just spent a couple of years doing a stint in the Army. But now I'm back, and I plan on staying. I stopped in to thank you."

"Thank me?"

"Yes—for something that happened several years ago, back in 1949." I recounted what had happened the night he discouraged me from letting him fill the prescription for the painkiller, and he nodded with the familiarity of a man recognizing a scenario that had occurred many times over the years. "I appreciated your complete honesty with me that day, even though it meant the loss of a sale for you," I said. "You were really concerned about me that day; you didn't want me to take anything that could potentially be harmful to me. That seemed to me to be pretty unusual for a businessman. I wanted to let you know just how much that incident affected my life." I went on to tell him how I was led into chiropractic because of it, adding, "Now I'm setting up my office not very far from here, at 5349½ West Belmont Avenue, just a couple of doors east of Long Avenue. We might even be seeing each other from time to time." Shaking his hand warmly, I said, "I want you to know that I will tell everyone what a wonderful person you are, and how I appreciated your honesty with me years ago. You may have lost a sale that night, but what you did changed the course of my life, and I will never forget it."

He thanked me for saying this, and I could see by the look in his eyes that he was touched by my words. Over the course of time, I have related the story of this honest pharmacist to many of my patients. Since my office was located less than a mile from his drugstore, I am convinced many of my patients also started doing business with him. People often feel keen loyalty to their pharmacists, and they want a pharmacist they can trust. Walter Kopec was a man who merited such respect, and I'm sure his honesty and sincere concern for the welfare of his customers helped in his success. He exemplified what life should be in the health care field—helping your fellow man and doing the very best you can at all times, with honesty and objectivity.

I also stopped by St. Stanislaus Roman Catholic Church. Both of my parents had long been members of that parish, and I also had been a member there for most of my life. It seemed to me a natural place to go, now that I was setting up my practice nearby, to ask the priest to place an announcement in the weekly church bulletin to let the congregation know that I had opened an office.

It now seems ironic to me that it was in this Polish Roman Catholic church that I had my earliest experience with antichiropractic prejudice. The priest hesitated, then haltingly said he would have to see if he would be allowed to publish the announcement. When I pressed him for an explanation, he said that chiropractic was unproved, and that the church's position on such matters was that it could not appear to endorse a healing art that the medical profession did not recognize. I respected his candor about caution, and I patiently explained the legitimacy of chiropractic and its recognition by the laws of the state of Illinois. I felt it was necessary to clarify the fact that organized medicine did not have governmental authority, and that therefore it was not the province of medical doctors to either legitimize or disenfranchise any alternative health care choice. The priest was unmoved. He said he would have to check with a church member who was a medical doctor and get his opinion. I asked for the name of the M.D. who would pass this judgment, and the priest gave it to me.

I visited the doctor's office to speak to him personally. During our brief conversation, he questioned why the church would ask him about this, and said it was not his place to pass judgment. He was evasive about giving approval of any kind. We were not discussing philosophies or patient referrals here; this was simply an issue of placing an announcement in a local church bulletin concerning the new enterprise of one of the church's members. After a couple more visits with the priest, I realized that he would not place the statement for me, and I gave up on the idea of a bulletin announcement.

Even with that minor discouragement, I did not realize what a honeymoon I was enjoying as I opened my office in the summer of 1955. I had waited so long to begin a professional life, and now I loved what I was doing, believed in it completely, and devoted myself wholeheartedly to establishing myself professionally and building my practice. Chiropractic is more than a vital profession. To me, and to many other doctors of chiropractic, it touches every waking hour and gives purpose and meaning to life. It is, in fact, a way of life. Some of us live, eat, and breathe chiropractic.

I was in debt when I opened my practice, and I invested in only the barest necessities. My parents generously assisted me with a loan to help me buy the necessary office equipment. I had no receptionist, and I had no professional associate, either, in those early days; I staffed my office entirely by myself. My biggest concerns were those common to all people starting out in business—being able to pay the rent and to meet monthly operating expenses.

When my practice was just getting started, there were not enough appointments to fill the day or to pay the rent, so I worked with my father during the mornings for the first year. My parents had sold the grocery business, but my dad continued to work as a painter, wallpaper-hanger, and decorator. I helped him for four hours a day, working until noon. Then I would go home for lunch, make a quick change, and head for my office to start seeing patients at two o'clock. This year was a great experience for me personally because I really got to know my father better during the hours we spent together. It also gave my practice time to begin growing.

The 1950s were not a period of great negativism toward chiropractic. If there were disapproving comments of any kind, they focused on the idea that chiropractic was a young, upstart profession that was not scientifically proved. Public knowledge of chiropractic was relatively limited, and the general attitude toward chiropractic as a health care alternative was largely indifferent. Most public education about chiropractic was initiated by chiropractors themselves, and there was no training program available to help chiropractors communicate information with expertise. I felt that the public was simply late in accepting the principles that made chiropractic achieve such excellent results, and that eventually public knowledge would catch up with what we already understood to be true.

At this time, some chiropractors were developing professional relationships with medical doctors, in terms of both communication and patient referrals, and with increasing frequency, M.D.s were even using the services of chiropractors. There was growing mutual respect and interprofessional cooperation between an increasing number of medical doctors and chiropractors. Compared with what was to follow in the 1960s, our professional existence was peaceful and very quiet.

In 1957, I joined my practice with that of Dr. Amon Hopf, which was at the intersection of Milwaukee Avenue and Pulaski Road, roughly a mile east of where my first office had been. He had a second-floor office across the hall from a bowling alley, and it was a noisy place. In the evenings we would hear excited screaming every time some bowler got a strike. Even so, this arrangement offered me amenities that I rather enjoyed; besides a colleague, there was also a receptionist, a luxury I had never had in my first office. Our professional collaboration was brief, however. Dr. Hopf passed away in 1958. I took over his office alone when he died.

In the meantime, I was able to relax a little more, as my practice was growing and doing well, and I was interested in having more of a private life. I like to dance, so for enjoyment, I went once a week to the dances at the Holiday Ballroom on the northwest side of Chicago. It was not long before I was regarded as a regular patron there, and I knew the others who attended regularly as well. One night a new, attractive face among a more familiar group of women caught my eye.

Ardith was a petite brunette, five feet two inches tall and well proportioned. She had a sweet face, and kind, gentle eyes. Interested in meeting and learning more about her, I asked her for a dance.

I liked Ardith immediately. She told me she was living with her mother, who had been a widow since Ardith's father had died of a sudden heart attack when Ardith was twelve years old. Ardith was a nice person with wholesome ideas, and as we talked, I recognized other commendable qualities as well. She was frugal and had worked to put herself through school to become a nurse. More important than her physical attractiveness was an inner beauty that I recognized almost immediately.

In the weeks that followed, we spent more and more time together, and in addition to my romantic interest in her, my admiration for Ardith also grew. I learned that she was already a registered nurse on a crack surgical team. She was working with Dr. Willis J. Potts, who had achieved national renown for having devised a surgical technique for the treatment of "blue babies." This surgical procedure redirected the flow of blood to the lungs so that the blood could be oxygenated, thereby correcting the blue baby phenomenon. Dr. Potts was chief of surgery and research at Chicago's Children's Memorial Hospital. He was a man who, despite having big hands, performed the most delicate surgical procedures on tiny newborns, with slow, meticulous precision. Ardith enjoyed her work as a surgical scrub nurse and was proud to say that, to her knowledge, no baby had ever died on the operating table when Dr. Potts was performing the surgery.

I shared with Ardith my dream of someday building a chiropractic clinic that would be the best example of what chiropractic can do. She admired me for having a goal in life beyond settling into a nine-to-five routine. It was not important to either of us that I make a lot of money, but it did matter that I contribute to society by helping people and working to make our world a better place.

Ardith and I were married on July 9, 1961, eight months after we first met. We made our first home together in an apartment conveniently located less than a block south of the office I had taken over from Dr. Hopf. I had only to cross the street to get to my office. For Ardith, however, the commute to Children's Hospital took over an hour. Although she loved working there, Ardith knew that as a nurse with her skills and experience, she could get a job in virtually any hospital. So she left the surgical team at Children's Memorial and took a position at a community hospital located closer to home. And there she experienced the real world of hospital medicine. She'd seen the best, and now she saw another side.

Reality had a brutal impact on her. After her first day on the job, Ardith came home in tears, saying she would never set foot in that hospital again! She noted that the surgical techniques were not even close to the standards she was accustomed to, indeed took for granted, at Children's Hospital. She had over-heard doctors talking about the money they were collecting as though it carried more weight with them than the medical serv-ices they were rendering. Until then, Ardith had put physicians on a pedestal, assuming they were all as conscientious and above reproach as those she worked with at Children's Hospital. Now she began to see them as no better or worse than any other group of people—perhaps no different even from used-car salesmen, who were widely considered the craftiest con artists in those days. Certainly these doctors were nothing like Dr. Potts!

I persuaded Ardith to stay in her new job and work to make it a better place. She did, but for her the bubble had burst, and hospital medicine never had the same respect in her mind as it had had before. Her love of professional nursing had not dimin-ished, and neither did she reject medicine and healing, but she was disillusioned by the selfish motivations and the mercenary mentality of the hospital and some of its healers. Before long, she reduced her hours at the hospital, working there primarily on weekends, and she became invaluable to me in yet another way—as the regular assistant in my chiropractic office.

2

A CLOUD
OF PROPAGANDA

I n the early 1960s, just as chiropractic was beginning to experience a surge of public popularity, the climate shifted quite suddenly. An unexpected onslaught of published material maligning chiropractic started coming from a wide variety of sources. This was both embarrassing and humiliating, and it chilled public recognition and acceptance of chiropractic as a legitimate healing profession.

It seemed to start sometime in late 1963. This new antagonism extended far beyond a lack of understanding of chiropractic or a refusal to take chiropractic seriously; this was outright hostility aimed specifically at our profession. The change in the environment created confusion within the chiropractic profession. Chiropractors were surprised, and we were divided as to what to do in response. As the 1960s continued, the attacks grew increasingly vicious. In fact, it seemed that the more successes chiropractic accomplished—not only with patients, but also with clinical studies and professional development—the more outlandish, offensive, and outrageous were the attacks against the profession.

Everything about chiropractic came under fire. While some of the charges had an element of truth at their core, it was inevitably twisted to cast a shadow on the profession as a whole. Other claims were totally fabricated. The underlying intent of all of it seemed to be to create public fear and distrust of chiropractic.

In the first place, attacks against the profession referred to chiropractic as a cult or a myth. In fact, the phrase, "unscientific cult," was used so often in this literature that chiropractic was rarely mentioned without it. That was the first clue, a proverbial red flag, that would alert us within the profession to the propagandist nature of the writing. Allegations of cultism understandably frightened away potential patients who had no previous experience with chiropractic philosophy or methods. Articles were written that portrayed chiropractic as some kind of mystical, questionable therapy that achieved results only in the minds of cult followers.

Second, when chronic sufferers who were unresponsive to medical care found relief after a course of chiropractic treatments, their experiences were discounted in the literature as cases in which an affliction "ran its course." It was alleged that the results chiropractors were achieving were either purely chance occurrences—the problems would have gotten better anyway—or signs that the ailments had been psychosomatic in the first place. Incredibly, it was asserted that chiropractors just talked patients into feeling better. Bear in mind that many people had suffered for long periods of time, in some cases for many years, with very real ailments, because they received either ineffectual medical care or no care at all. Because they needed and chose to obtain chiropractic care, they were painted as gullible, brainwashed unfortunates who gave undeserved credit to chiropractors for their cures when (so asserted the propaganda) they just happened to get better after the cause of their distress ran its course. (Meanwhile, we must have been the luckiest doctors around, because so many of our patients' physical ailments just happened to "run their course" right after the patients began receiving chiropractic treatments.)

This second line of propaganda was then tied into the first, and used as evidence that the profession was indeed an "unscientific cult." Questions were raised—sometimes implied, but often stated outright—regarding the basis of chiropractic, and whether or not the practice was sound and scientifically based. It was suggested that the quality of chiropractic colleges was inferior, and that the profession's doctors, ethics, and modalities of treatment were substandard. There has long been a misconception that chiropractic is not scientifically based; in truth, it is more scientifically sound within its realm of health care than many other disciplines of modern medicine are. Another attack on the educational background of chiropractors concerned the very origin of chiropractic. For example, the first chiropractor was referred to as a "fish peddler," with the clear implication that no health care profession emerging from such roots could possibly have credibility or merit. In truth, the first chiropractor was a grocer, and he probably did sell some fish, but let us then recognize also that the first surgeons were barbers and bloodletters—George Washington died after being bled by one of them—and that the original M.D.s were not men of science at all, but merely itinerant peddlers who traveled around in wagons promoting worthless and even dangerous remedies and drugs.[1] But truth, apparently, was not the issue. The point was to create prejudice, ignorance, and fear of anything that was not medical. (*See* The Relative Safety of Chiropractic on page 30.)

Finally, there were allegations that chiropractors claimed chiropractic could cure anything. This was patently absurd. Some of the early writings of Dr. Daniel David Palmer, the founder of chiropractic, had implied that he believed all disease had a single cause, and therefore that one type of treatment could cure any ailment. However, the chiropractic profession had long since abandoned this single cause/single cure theory of disease, and any reading of modern chiropractic literature would have shown this. Nor did chiropractic deny the role of bacteria, viruses, and other microorganisms in human illness. In fact, the study of bacteriology is a requirement in the curriculum of every chiropractic college in America.

Medical textbooks frequently discuss *predisposing causes* and *exciting causes* of disease. A weakened immune system, which renders the body more vulnerable to infection, is an example of a predisposing cause; viruses and bacteria, which take hold of the body and directly cause illness, are examples of exciting causes. Vertebral subluxations, which impede the proper functioning of the nerves, result in lowered tissue resistance, and are therefore a predisposing cause of disease. By treating subluxations, a chiropractor helps the body to raise its own natural resistance, so that it is less likely to fall victim to the exciting causes of illness. Thus chiropractic and orthodox medicine both subscribe to the basic principle of exciting and predisposing causes of disease, but while orthodox medicine primarily intervenes to combat the exciting causes, chiropractic focuses on removing the predisposing causes.

The Relative Safety
of Chiropractic

Medical propagandists have often attempted to discredit chiro-
practic by repeating lies about it. One example is the allegation
that chiropractic is dangerous—specifically, that chiropractic
adjustments can cause strokes. In truth, many factors can bring
on a stroke, including climbing a flight of stairs, becoming emo-
tionally upset as a result of an argument, worrying, having
indigestion, taking medications, or even engaging in sexual in-
tercourse. In many cases, strokes occur with no obvious causative
factors at all, such as during sleep.

The risk of serious complications from spinal manipulation of the
neck was studied by Dr. Andreis Kleynhans, head of a chiropractic
college in Australia. An exhaustive study of medical literature
spanning a period of thirty-one years (1947 to 1978), during which
billions of chiropractic adjustments were performed, found a total of
ten cases of death from stroke following spinal manipulation. Nine
of these followed manipulation by medical doctors. Only one oc-
curred following chiropractic adjustment.[1] The obvious message
here would seem to be that spinal adjusting should be done only by
chiropractors, who have superior skill and understanding of such
manipulation. Government commissions have concluded that chiro-
practic training is far more sophisticated and better designed than
the courses taught in physical therapy schools or weekend courses
for medics who dabble in manipulation.[2]

A separate study by Paul Jaskoviak, D.C., at the National
College of Chiropractic in Lombard, Illinois, concurred that the
risk of stroke has been exaggerated beyond reasonable limits by
medical propagandists. He found that of an estimated 5 million
adjustments, given for the most part by students at the college,
not one has ever caused a vertebral artery injury and stroke.[3]

Other researchers have calculated the chance of a stroke follow-
ing chiropractic adjustment to be between 1 in 1 million and
1 in 20 million.[4] Furthermore, it is questionable that many

of the reported cases of stroke that followed spinal manipulation were actually caused by the manipulation. With over 50,000 chiropractors practicing in America, the sheer numbers both of professionals and of adjustments done every day make it likely that a person who suffers a stroke might coincidentally have had a chiropractic adjustment a day or two earlier.

Moreover, to put these numbers into perspective, medical doctors would love to have such statistics on their side. In fact, a comparison of people receiving different types of treatment for neck pain over the course of one year found that the incidence of complications among people taking nonsteroidal anti-inflammatory drugs (NSAIDs) such as aspirin or ibuprofen was 100 times higher than that among people receiving cervical (neck) manipulation treatments, and that the risk of death was 400 times higher in the NSAID group.[5] Thus, while NSAIDs are widely recognized as safe treatments for many disorders, it is fair to say that spinal manipulation is hundreds of times safer. Put in proper perspective, then, the risk of stroke following chiropractic adjustment cannot be viewed as a reasonable concern.

While it might have been simple and possible to deal with one or two of these general areas of criticism, thereby effectively putting to rest any serious doubts created in the minds of people who read the literature, the incredible amount of misinformation coming from so many directions at one time confounded anyone wanting to attempt to dispel the lies that were being created. It was unclear how we might reasonably and appropriately cope with the assaults now striking at every facet of chiropractic. Initially, the chiropractic profession thought it best to exercise patience and tolerance, and to have no visible reaction. We hoped the disturbance was nothing more than a momentary storm destined to blow over and be done. But chiropractors also did not know how to fight back. Angry, frustrated chiropractors wrote articles for chiropractic journals protesting the inaccuracies of the propaganda, but these served no meaningful purpose, as only chiropractors read them.

Meanwhile, articles attacking chiropractic appeared in newspapers, magazines, and newsletters from all over the country.

Incredibly, however, the material from these widely divergent sources all sounded quite similar. There began to be a commonality, in fact a characteristic ring, to all this material. The phrases, clichés, and cases cited as examples began to echo one another.

As a professional, I attended meetings and conventions of both the state and national chiropractic associations. Often at these gatherings I asked other chiropractors if they, as individual practitioners, subscribed to the bizarre "cure-all" claims and other outrageous beliefs that the media were ascribing to chiropractic professionals. Not once did I find a chiropractor who did. (If I had, I certainly would have confronted him or her about such radical claims, and I would have made such an individual understand that he or she did not represent the majority.) This is not to say that I did not believe there were a few irrational chiropractors who believe that chiropractic heals every ailment known to man—among over 50,000 people in any profession, some peculiar dissidents can be found. But neither I nor any of my colleagues knew of or could find such a person. This teaching had not been part of any of our original chiropractic training. Perhaps more importantly, individuals who believed it did not attend the professional seminars.

A statistical study concluded in 1963 by Batten and Associates surveyed over 6,000 chiropractors throughout the United States and Canada, and determined that over 90 percent of them had referred, and continued to refer, patients who needed medical care to doctors of medicine.[2] On the other hand, the progress made in the 1950s in chiropractor/medical doctor cooperation had reversed by the mid-1960s, so that in virtually every case, M.D.s had ceased to refer to chiropractors those patients they believed would have fared better under chiropractic care. If any group was guilty of having a cure-all attitude regarding its own philosophy of healing, it was clearly the medical practitioners.

Still, newspapers across the United States and Canada persisted in printing articles blasting the practice of chiropractic, as did news magazines and journals of medicine. There is something exceedingly ominous about misrepresentations that are printed in black and white. The reader naïvely tends to believe that whatever is printed is intended to protect and enlighten us, and therefore must indeed be true—that our laws prevent libelous lies from being published. Lies and innuendoes are difficult to challenge directly; written rebuttals most often are not regarded by publishers as being of interest to readers, and therefore are not published—or, if they do make it into print, they are generally relegated to some back section of the newspaper as space-fillers. The allegations themselves, infinitely more sensational in nature, make splashier headlines.

The negative propaganda became so predictable that I would no sooner begin reading an article than I could recognize what it was going to say and how it would make its case. All of the "information" these pieces contained fell into one or more of seven categories:

1. *Innuendoes*—statements implying or suggesting a wrongdoing by a chiropractor that, if challenged, could not be supported by fact.

2. *Material taken out of context* to create an image worse than or different from reality by removing key facts surrounding an issue.

3. *Half-truths*—portions of truth manipulated so as to create false impressions or conclusions, never telling the whole story.

4. *Obsolete material* that represented outdated statements of earlier chiropractors as the thinking of modern chiropractic.

5. *Obscure sources* that were cited as authoritative—such as random, bizarre comments made by some unknown or obscure chiropractor that were used to hold all within the profession up to ridicule and embarrassment.

6. *Incidental exceptions* to the rule presented as commonplace occurrences.

7. *Outright lies*—the same tactic Nazi propagandists had used more than twenty years earlier on the principle that the more outrageous the falsehood, the more believable it becomes.

To compound an already bad situation, in 1967 the state of Illinois was among a number of states that began enforcing "ethics laws" that made it illegal for doctors to advertise their services. These laws did not extend to drug manufacturers, who were free to spend money lavishly to promote drugs as the best approach to many health problems—some of which, credible clinical results had proved, could have been better treated

through natural chiropractic methods. Given the freedom that
the pharmaceutical companies continued to enjoy in advertising
their products, these ethics laws effectively created a two-
pronged support of organized medicine. On the one hand, the
drug companies were free to advertise the effectiveness of pills
and medicinal health care for different sorts of ailments, while
chiropractors faced the possibility of having their licenses re-
voked for unlawful advertising if they signed their names to any
attempt to defend or advocate for their profession in the media.
On the other hand, the antichiropractic propaganda had a negative impact on chiropractic. The endorsement of this situation by
many medical doctors seemed obvious to me, although at the
time I concluded that most M.D.s must be either misguided or
simply unaware of the truth about chiropractic.

We did not know what was precipitating the onslaught of
attacks against chiropractic, but many different individuals, organizations, and publications seemed to be involved, including
state legislatures. The ethics laws may have sounded well inten-
tioned on the surface, but they effectively suppressed chiropractors from informing the public about the advantages chiropractic offers.*

At the time all of this was going on, I had been writing a
weekly educational health column in a local Polish-language
newspaper for about ten years. Many of the people in the area
had immigrated to this country from Poland, and if they were
ignorant of chiropractic, at least they were not prejudiced
against it. I was tapping a whole new group of people, and my
only barrier was ignorance, not prejudice. But suddenly I received a notice from the Illinois Board of Examiners saying that
I must immediately stop writing my articles or risk losing my
state license to practice chiropractic. It would have been professional suicide for me to challenge this ultimatum on my own,
but I felt that the state chiropractic society should have challenged it as unconstitutional and discriminatory. The Illinois

---

*Eventually the federal court ruled that prohibiting the communication of
information, even on supposedly ethical grounds, was a violation of the
right to free speech, and ultimately the Supreme Court ruled these laws
unconstitutional. But while these laws were in effect, they crippled the
dissemination of the chiropractic message.

Chiropractic Society, however, refused to do so. For about a year I discontinued the column, until finally the word came down that the Supreme Court had found the ethics laws to be unconstitutional.

During this time it became common in antichiropractic propaganda to dwell on the indiscretions and lack of professionalism of a few chiropractors, and to portray them as representing all chiropractic practitioners. Certain isolated cases received far more attention than they deserved. One case that came to the media's attention dated back to 1961 and involved a young girl who had had a cancerous tumor of the eye. A chiropractor in California had continued to treat her, instead of referring her for medical care appropriate to her condition, and the little girl succumbed to the cancer. Clearly, this chiropractor was seriously out of line. But this case seemed to resurface for years in various newspaper and magazine articles, with no regard for a balanced viewpoint. Few isolated cases of medical malpractice have ever been used and reused to the extent that this case was. It was repeated over and over for a period of years as a basis for maligning an entire profession.

In the second half of the 1960s, incidents echoing the antichiropractic propaganda dealt blows to the profession. In 1967, the United States Congress was considering the demands of independent licensed healing professions to be included among those covered by Medicare, professions that included chiropractic, optometry, and occupational therapy, among others. This provided the opportunity for the Congress to suggest that the government conduct a study of the need for and cost of covering licensed nonmedical practitioners.

Such a study was ordered in the 1967 amendments to the Social Security Act, and the U.S. Department of Health, Education, and Welfare (HEW) appointed two committees to prepare an HEW study report.* The first of these was the Ad Hoc Consultant Group for the Independent Professions; it consisted of twenty-two people, including seven M.D.s, one osteopath, one

---

*In addition to chiropractors, eight other types of independent practitioners were selected for inclusion in the HEW study, among them audiologists, corrective therapists, physical therapists, psychologists, social workers, and speech pathologists.

hospital administrator, one nursing service official, and others—
but not a single chiropractor. This group was responsible to John
Cashman, Assistant Surgeon General, who by his own admission was opposed to chiropractic before the study began. The
second committee was the Expert Review Panel for Chiropractic,
Naturopathy, and Naprapathy, made up of eight members, five
of whom were M.D.s and one of whom was a medical school
official—but again, no chiropractors. The medical orientation of
both of these committees was virtually guaranteed to give them
a professional and institutional bias against chiropractic from
the outset. Furthermore, the members of the group were not
permitted even to visit a chiropractic college in the course of
their investigations.[3]

The study itself was a disaster. The study's report presented
biased misstatements about chiropractic and called them facts,
was grossly inadequate and erroneous in its information, and
did not confine itself to the specific purpose of need and costs.
The HEW report was sent to the Congress in December 1968.[4] It
was the most hard-hitting denial yet of chiropractic as a health
care service. The AMA called it a victory, touting it as "an
unbiased, independent government agency report that rejected
chiropractic."[5]

The American Chiropractic Association, the International
Chiropractors Association, and the Council of State Chiropractic
Examining Boards were outraged by this partial study and biased report. In response, they jointly authored a white paper in
May 1969 protesting the lack of chiropractic representation on
the two committees, exposing the AMA's heavy hand in the
study, and firmly maintaining that it was in the public interest
to include coverage for chiropractic in the Medicare program.
The chiropractic organizations agreed that chiropractic had to
remain a separate and distinct healing profession, and that while
drugs and surgery had merit, they did not belong within the
scope of chiropractic's therapy.

On the heels of the HEW study, the January 1969 issue of
Senior Citizens News, a periodical published by the National
Council of Senior Citizens (NCSC), included an article that was
full of the same propaganda and misinformation we had been
seeing elsewhere. Under the heading "Why Chiropractic Cult
Cannot Provide Quality Health Care," it stated: "The National

Council of Senior Citizens, in specific resolutions approved by large majorities of delegates attending its annual conventions, has continued to urge that the services of chiropractors be barred from coverage under the Medicare program."[6] This article blasted chiropractic with many of the well-known clichés, and said that the National Council for Senior Citizens "stood solidly with . . . organized medicine in condemning chiropractic as an unscientific cult."[7] It was a classic propaganda piece, echoing thought for thought, and in some places word for word, the propaganda that had been spread by individuals we increasingly began to recognize as mouthpieces of organized medicine. Among the statements made in the *Senior Citizens News* article was this: "With chiropractic and other completely unscientific cults, there is no possibility for quality health care."[8]

The NCSC boasted 2,500,000 members, and its publication was very far-reaching. Even though the article was published during the campaign by organized medicine to prevent chiropractic services from being covered under Medicare, it came as a surprise to the chiropractic profession. Only the year before, in 1968, the NCSC Social Security Committee had recommended adopting a resolution that chiropractic care be covered under Medicare, but the organization's executive committee had postponed the vote on the resolution that year. In 1969, they suppressed delegates from bringing it to the floor. The NCSC executive committee, in effect, worked against the interests of its own members, the majority of whom were recipients of Medicare via Social Security, and the NCSC became one of the leading forces advocating the exclusion of chiropractic health care coverage. The *Senior Citizens News* article, which was presented as an independent report coming from outside medicine, was used extensively and given wide distribution by the AMA as that organization presented its so-called evidence against chiropractic. It was a major blow based entirely upon false information, and its impact was felt most effectively on the political front, especially on Capitol Hill.

Shortly after the blasting by the NCSC newspaper, the Health Insurance Association of America (HIAA) issued a policy statement that suggested excluding limited practitioners (health care practitioners who are restricted by law to a particular form of therapy) from private health care coverage plans.[9] The HIAA is a trade association for hundreds of private insurance companies and, as the policy-making group for the health insurance industry, has a significant influence on those companies. Any policy formulated by this association is likely to be adopted by its member organizations. This policy statement was carefully worded so as not to specifically name chiropractic, but it used as supporting documentation the December 1968 HEW report, and it effectively injured insurance company relations with chiropractors.

The policy statement in question, dated February 19, 1969, stated that "manipulative services and subluxations for the purpose of removing nerve interference" should be deleted from insurance coverage. Basically, by definition, this exclusion specifically extended to the services of chiropractors. Chiropractors protested the wording, but the HIAA simply said it had no control over how this statement was interpreted.

Then, in July 1969, a book entitled *At Your Own Risk: The Case Against Chiropractic* was published. Its author was Ralph Lee Smith, who had previously established himself as unfriendly to chiropractic with articles in the *National Enquirer* and other publications. The book offered the same argument, which it upheld as independent opinion, against coverage of chiropractic services under Medicare. Among the statements included in the book intended to shake public confidence in chiropractic was this: "In 1945, *Medical World News* reported that it was still possible to obtain a mail-order doctor of chiropractic degree from a Chicago college for $127.50."[10]

I contacted *Medical World News* to ask why it would have published such an outrageously false claim. Ronnie Mark, the records librarian of the publication, replied that she could find no record of their ever having made any such statement. Moreover, she said, *Medical World News* did not even exist in 1945! It was not published until 1960, fifteen years later.[11]

At this point it was becoming crystal clear that the negative messages were severely damaging the professional image of chiropractic, and that they were discouraging potential patients from choosing a form of health care that in many cases would have proved superior to the methods they were using. During this period, I would occasionally have patients cancel or simply not show up for appointments because they had been frightened by the negative propaganda they had heard. The propaganda was, in fact, so convincing that even I could see how people might be swayed by it.

There were, of course, faithful patients who continued in chiropractic therapy even as the barrage of attacks against it made it unpopular to do so, but even they frequently chose not to talk about it. One such patient candidly admitted to me that she lied to her friends and neighbors when she kept her appointments at my office. She said, "People laugh at me when I tell them I'm going to a chiropractor, so rather than be laughed at, I tell them I'm going shopping." Then she added encouragingly, "People are dumb, but what are you going to do?"

Chiropractors have an old saying: "People don't have to believe in chiropractic to get results." Throughout this time, in the face of all the negative propaganda, chiropractors quietly continued to effect amazing results with patients.

As it was becoming clear that the barrage of propaganda was hurting chiropractors, it was also becoming obvious that the similarities in all the attacks were in no way coincidental. But who could be responsible? It was a mystery how, and by whom, these attacks from all sides could have been coordinated. The assaults on chiropractic were so effective that I sensed the effort must be an organized one. I believed that whoever was responsible for the profuse amount of hostile material must be a misguided, bigoted group—perhaps people so blindly prejudiced that they could not recognize the truth. The effect of the misinformation they were spreading appeared to be intended to create more blind prejudice, and to ensure that people would not see the truth about chiropractic. And the more accomplishments chiropractic achieved, the more hostile the attacks became. Oliver Wendell Holmes once wrote, "The mind of the bigot is like the pupil of the eye: the more light you pour upon it, the more it will contract.[12] This described exactly what I saw happening. It would be several years, however, before the full picture of what was really going on, and of the central source of this onslaught, would come clearly into focus.

* * *

As the 1960s drew to a close, it had become clear that quiet tolerance on the part of chiropractic was not accomplishing anything, and my patience had worn thin for the propaganda to end. Chiro-practic needed to respond by mobilizing those within the pro-fession to become more vocal as a group. I passionately believed, even early in my career, that my profession had long been too soft toward its adversaries, and that we needed to unite in an assertive education program to enlighten the public about the truth. I realized that a rational, systematic effort on the part of chiropractors would be required if we were ever to make the public understand the sensible basis of the chiropractic point of view. How this might be done, however, I had not yet resolved in my own mind.

Chiropractors represented a minority group of solid citizens who contributed in a major way to improving the quality of life of those they touched. There were only two groups of people who would promote chiropractic: patients who were grateful for the results they had found with chiropractic (and they have always been the real strength behind the success of the profession), and chiropractors themselves, who quietly performed their miracles every day. Nei-ther group was inclined to go to the media to make its case and rally public support for chiropractic. And public support was what the profession needed. As Abraham Lincoln once said, "Public opinion is everything. With public sentiment nothing can fail; without it nothing can succeed."[13]

Then, in 1970, Dr. Leonard Fay of the National College of Chiropractic in Chicago launched a program to teach communi-cations skills to chiropractors. He planned to have one meeting a month for twelve months, with material provided to be studied (and added to) between classes. This was great! I was thrilled and inspired by the concept of the program, which to my way of thinking was long overdue. As it happened, this series of meetings would totally transform my professional life over the course of the next year, and would begin to redirect my destiny.

This is not to say that I was eager to become a public speaker. I was intimidated by the very thought of standing before a crowd of people. But I believed that speaking out was necessary in order to fight this battle. Chiropractic needed willing and capa-ble spokespeople, and I prepared to confront my fears head on.

As early as the first meeting, it became clear that there was no published material available covering the vast amount of back-ground and rebuttal information that one would need to speak successfully to the media about the issues confronting chiropractic. I asked why our profession did not have a resource of that kind, since it was so desperately needed to counteract the barrage of negative propaganda against us. Dr. Fay explained that it would take a great deal of research, time, and money in order to compile into a single text the comprehensive information needed. Then and there I decided that I would compile the notes myself for such a reference book, realizing it would take over a year to do it.

The meetings were exciting. I was so turned on by the meetings that when they broke up, I would forego the social hour and pizza with the other doctors—I couldn't get home fast enough to organize and develop the material gathered that evening. My schedule was conveniently arranged so that I didn't have office hours the following day, and I would work at home through the night on my project. I was convinced the result of it would be a resource that would be the answer to chiropractic's dilemma. I hopefully imagined that as we educated the public to see the light regarding our profession, the antichiropractic propagandists would also come to accept us, and even that we might finally become coworkers with medical doctors for the benefit of our patients.

After eagerly attending every one of Dr. Fay's meetings during that twelve-month period, and reading every antichiropractic article I could find, I had accumulated and analyzed a massive amount of information. I compiled everything into a loose-leaf notebook that was about three inches thick. I had gathered notes containing rebuttals to all of the negative propaganda that kept surfacing at that time. My notes were so thorough that I felt there was nothing an adversary could say that I could not counter. With this data complete, I investigated ways to put it into manuscript form for other interested chiropractors to use. I felt it would be important for copies of the accumulated information to be made available for anyone interested in approaching broadcasters and newspapers, and speaking publicly about the wonders of chiropractic. The information could also potentially be useful to chiropractors for patient education classes and, if necessary, in preparing courtroom testimony.

One of my patients worked for a major publishing company. He reviewed my manuscript and concluded it would make a compelling book. He brought it to the attention of his company and attempted to persuade the editors to publish it, but my book was out of their realm; they did not publish books on subjects relating to health or medicine. Encouraged rather than disheartened, I decided to publish the book privately. My patient suggested I modify the manuscript, writing in layman's terms to create a book for the general market. That way, chiropractors could learn from the facts included in the material and, at the same time, the public could also be educated. Thus, quite by accident, what initially had been intended as a public speaking resource for chiropractors was transformed into a book suitable for the broader general market.

The book was entitled *Chiropractic Speaks Out—A Reply to Medical Propaganda, Bigotry and Ignorance.* By the time it was first published, early in 1973, I had reason to believe that the subtitle defined much of the problem. The text exposed what I had come to understand as a deliberate attempt to slander and subvert the chiropractic profession.

Because I published the book independently, it was not realistic for me to try to sell it in bookstores. They would want the book on consignment, and then if the books did not sell, they would return them, possibly damaged and not saleable, which would have been a bookkeeping and billing nightmare. To promote the book, I made myself available as a speaker for state chiropractic associations that were willing to make arrangements with radio or television programs, pay my transportation expenses, and buy some books. During the program, I would make it known that the books were available from local chiropractors, who became the booksellers.

* * *

Quite coincidentally, in 1972, shortly before my book was published, another book came out. The name of this book was *In the Public Interest,* and its author was William Trever. It created quite a stir in chiropractic circles because of allegations it contained of improper conduct by influential leaders within the American Medical Association. Unfortunately, the book received little attention outside the chiropractic profession.

It is interesting—and it was indeed no accident—how the

Trever book initially got into the hands of people within the chiropractic profession. Sellers of the book covertly contacted the American Chiropractic Association (ACA), the larger of the two national professional associations, and offered them the opportunity to purchase the book. They were referred to the ACA's legal counsel and Washington lobbyist, Harry Rosenfield. He responded with no interest whatsoever, so, perhaps slightly discouraged, the group turned to the smaller professional chiropractic organization, the International Chiropractors Association (ICA). The response there was entirely different. The ICA agreed to purchase the entire stock of books. The sellers demanded, as terms for the sale, that they be able to arrive unannounced with a truckload of books, make a quick drop-off of volumes, receive payment by means of a cashier's check for $2,500, and then quickly disappear. But before the sellers of the book vanished, the ICA purchased the rights to the copyrighted material, and with it permission to reprint the book or portions of it if they chose to do so.

In the Public Interest had been printed by an underground press identified in the book as Scriptures Unlimited, whose address was given as an already-closed post office box in Los Angeles, California. "William Trever" was a pseudonym. A statement inside the book claimed that it had been made possible through the assistance of a group called the Reform in Professional Organizations Freedom Foundation. It was probably no accident that those initials spelled RIPOFF.

The book's original cover depicted the AMA's caduceus (serpent-on-the-staff) emblem superimposed on a Nazi-style swastika. The book's tone was sarcastic, and it contained a number of offensive illustrations (sketches similar to political cartoon satire) that were insulting to the AMA. My initial reaction was that the book was trash and ought to be tossed in the wastebasket. Fortunately, I did not dismiss the book quite so quickly. It was a real shocker.

It quickly became clear why the sellers of this book had felt it would be of particular interest to the chiropractic professional organizations. With an abundance of what was alleged to be authentic documentation, it supported some facts already outlined within my own book, and it also opened my eyes to the fact that the framers of the antichiropractic propaganda were not merely ignorant, biased, or prejudiced; more than that, they were arrogantly dishonest, systematic, and vicious in their smear campaign against chiropractic. The book pointedly identified the ultimate perpetrators of this false information as being none other than powerful leadership within the American Medical Association—namely, H. Doyl Taylor and Robert Throckmorton, who were both attorneys; Joseph A. Sabatier, Jr., and H. Thomas Ballantine, both medical doctors; and others.

The American public tends to put the AMA on something of a pedestal. The organization's very name implies that the AMA concerns itself with everything medical and health related, even though it does not. But the public seems to believe that it does, and that in order for chiropractic to be a legitimate healing art, the AMA must somehow officially recognize it. The reality is that the only forms of recognition that matter are being licensed by the states—which chiropractors are; having a federally approved accrediting agency for educational institutions—which chiropractic does; and being covered by most insurance companies, Medicare, and Medicaid—which chiropractic care is.

Part of the public confusion over the role of the American Medical Association stems from the conduct of the AMA itself, which often represents itself as acting in the public's interest—as though it has been entrusted with that interest. In fact, the AMA is nothing more than a private trade organization representing the collective interests of its members, who are medical doctors. It is not the province of any trade association to recognize or to support any interest other than its own. Yet there is a lingering misperception that the AMA has a special interest in and authority over everything relating to health care.

As I got deeper into reading *In the Public Interest,* I found the book to be intelligently written, and the information it contained to be abundantly documented by what appeared to be photocopies of internal memoranda and other correspondence that had been smuggled out of the headquarters of the American Medical Association. AMA headquarters, located in Chicago, is a heavily guarded structure. Security there is extremely tight. Guards and video cameras are everywhere. Everyone needs an identification badge to get past the guards at the entrance, and no one is permitted to enter without appropriate credentials. Yet it looked as if somehow, someone had managed to smuggle an incredible amount of incriminating information out of the head-quarters for the compilation of this volume.

The secret internal documents and memos reproduced in this book for the first time shed light on an AMA master plan. They revealed that the AMA had organized and funded a special committee and, according to the book, called it the Committee on Quackery. Actually, the AMA Board of Trustees had first considered calling it the Committee on Chiropractic, but then they decided that this would dignify our profession.[14] It suited their purposes better to use the more negative terminology. This way their efforts could have a more benevolent sound—as though they were cleaning out the quacks within medicine. In reality, the AMA was deeply concerned about competition.

I came to a quote from a memorandum sent by from the Committee on Quackery to the AMA Board of Trustees. This document began:

> Since the AMA Board of Trustees' decision, at its meeting on November 2–3, 1963, to establish a Committee on Quackery, your Committee has considered its prime mission to be, first, the containment of chiropractic and, ultimately, the elimination of chiropractic.
>
> Your Committee believes it is well along in its first mission and is, at the same time, moving toward the ultimate goal. This, then, might be considered a progress report on developments in the past seven years. The Committee has not previously submitted such a report because it believes that to make public some of its activities would have been and continues to be unwise. Thus, this report is intended only for the information of the Board of Trustees.[15]

A cold chill of shock went through me. Here was a widely respected professional organization, one of the most powerful lobbying groups in the nation, actively working to eliminate me and my profession! And there was more. The secret internal documents and memos reproduced in this book contained evidence of exactly how the committee felt chiropractic could be eliminated as a competitor to medicine.

A number of documents showed how the AMA had planned to use an "ethical practices" mandate as a weapon against the chiropractic profession. Indeed, one of the first tasks undertaken by the Committee on Quackery had been to ensure that no medical doctors would associate professionally with chiropractors. Increasing numbers of M.D.s had begun to associate professionally with chiropractors as the 1950s progressed and the 1960s began. Apparently, the committee felt that this trend had to be stopped, and they planned to accomplish this by organizing a boycott preventing association by any members of the organized medical establishment with chiropractic interests or services. The mechanism was simple enough. First, the AMA adopted the position that none of its members could ethically associate with "unscientific cults." And then it declared chiropractic to be an unscientific cult. (*See* How Scientific Is Chiropractic?, page 47.)

As an internal AMA committee report that effectively summarized the purpose of the organization's master plan put it:

> [A]s recommended by your Committee and as submitted by the Board of Trustees, the AMA House of Delegates, for the first time, adopted a specific statement of policy on chiropractic.
>
> This was the necessary tool with which your committee has been able to widen the base of its chiropractic campaign. With it, other health-related groups were asked and did adopt the AMA policy statement or individually-phrased versions of it. These, in turn, led to even wider acceptance of the AMA position.[16]

The new AMA position, as given in an official policy statement adopted by the AMA House of Delegates at its clinical convention in November 1966, read as follows:

> It is the position of the medical profession that chiropractic is an unscientific cult whose practitioners lack the necessary training and background to diagnose and treat human disease. Chiropractic constitutes a hazard to rational health care in the United States because of the substandard and unscientific education of its practitioners and their rigid adherence to an irrational, unscientific approach to disease causation.[17]

The book went on to allege that the AMA had enlisted the support of other groups in order to implement the boycott.[18] One of these organizations was the Joint Commission on Accreditation of Hospitals (JCAH), a trade association made up of representatives of the AMA, the American Hospital Association,

How Scientific
Is Chiropractic?

According to "In the Public Interest," the AMA's definition of a "cult" was given in a memorandum that came out of the Department of Investigation headed by H. Doyl Taylor. A cult was defined as "a method based on the teaching (thoughts) of one man that is adhered to regardless of any scientific evidence to the contrary."[1]

The AMA had no scientific proof that what chiropractors were doing was wrong, yet they said chiropractic techniques were invalid. At the same time, they said, as recorded in the minutes of the January 9, 1967, meeting of the AMA's Committee on Quackery, that "many actual maneuvers used by chiropractors are quite similar to those used by physicians," referring to the manipulative techniques used by some osteopaths, orthopedic surgeons, and physiatrists.[2]

Science can be described as systematized knowledge derived from observation, study, and experimentation conducted in order to determine the nature of the thing being studied. With respect to chiropractic, researchers have applied specific types of treatments, called adjustments, to groups of people with certain ailments, and through carefully controlled studies have been able to achieve predictable results, to get them consistently, and to have both doctor (objectively) and patient (subjectively) agree that the treatments effected the desired improvement. This fulfills the requirements for scientific study. It does not mean that no further research is needed, but it does conclusively show that chiropractic is therapeutically effective. In fact, there are more randomized controlled studies that show the benefits of chiropractic, within its realm of health care, than there are for many of the therapies used by medical doctors.[3]

In 1992, the British Medical Journal published an editorial by Richard Smith concerning the research of Dr. David Eddy.[4] Among the findings cited are the following:

• *Only 15 percent of medical interventions have valid scientific basis or evidence. That means that 85 percent of medical treatments have no scientific basis or studies to support them.*

• *Only 1 percent of the articles in medical journals are scientifically sound.*

• *Many of the medical treatments utilized today have never been assessed at all.*[5]

As a cardiothoracic surgeon in Stanford, California, Dr. Eddy had become alarmed at the total lack of evidence to support the effectiveness of treatments he was using with patients. He identified glaucoma as an example of a condition with a medically well established treatment. Glaucoma is an ailment in which the pressure inside the eyeball increases to a dangerous level, and can result in progressive vision loss and, eventually, blindness. Therefore, when pressure rises beyond a certain level, physicians recommend treatment to lower it. This idea has simply been handed down from one generation to another, and while it is known that various treatments effectively lower the pressure, Dr. Eddy could not find any evidence of even a single controlled trial or study to support the belief that treatment to lower pressure actually was effective at halting vision loss.[6]

Dr. Eddy is a professor of health policy and management at Duke University in North Carolina, and is an advisor for the U.S. Agency for Health Care Policy and Research (AHCPR), a federal agency established in December 1989 to assist in the development and maintenance of national health practice guidelines. He is one of the most in-demand consultants on health standards and policy in the United States. He has taught courses to medical groups on how to reach consensus on the best medical management. For his study, he evaluated twenty-one areas of medical practice and judged the scientific studies of the effectiveness of treatments in seventeen of those areas as being "between poor and none . . . usually the best evidence was something less than a randomised controlled trial."[7] *The randomized controlled trial is in theory the most scientific method of testing the effectiveness of any health care treatment.*

> *Meanwhile, there are clinical and research data on the effectiveness of chiropractic that have come from studies done by prominent medical centers at major universities. There are also government studies; hospital studies; a study done by AV-MED, the largest health maintenance organization (HMO) in the southeastern United States; and a study done by RAND, a respected independent research group whose clients have included the United States government. Again and again, these studies show that chiropractic is indeed a safe, effective, and cost-efficient form of treatment, and that it can be more effective for low back pain than medical methods.[8]*

the American College of Surgeons, and the American College of Physicians. The JCAH agreed that none of its member hospitals was either to deal professionally with chiropractors or to include chiropractors as members of their medical staffs. If any did, it would risk having its hospital accreditation withdrawn or refused. A hospital lacking such accreditation could lose all of the accompanying benefits, such as residency programs, educational programs, and insurance programs—losses that, of course, would prove detrimental to the hospital. This put pressure on the hospitals to police the members of their medical staffs for compliance. An M.D. without hospital privileges would be financially and professionally ruined, so the pressure to comply was understandably intense. The extension of the boycott gave the committee additional muscle by which it could enforce M.D. cooperation.[19]

Other steps in the antichiropractic campaign, as expressed in a memorandum summarizing a meeting of the Committee on Quackery, included the following:

1) Doing everything within our power to see that chiropractic coverage under Title 18 of the Medicare Law is not obtained.

2) Doing everything within our power to see that recognition or listing by the U.S. Office of Education of a chiropractic accrediting agency is not achieved.

3) To encourage continued separation of the two national chiropractic associations.

4) To encourage state medical societies to take the initiative in
their state legislatures in regard to legislation that might affect
the practice of chiropractic.[20]

At the same time, the committee took steps to publicly discredit
the chiropractic profession wherever it could. Another memorandum referred to packets of propaganda literature stressing that
chiropractic was an unscientific cult—packets that were distributed to all the members of the U.S. Congress.[21] There was mention
of the possibility of public service announcements for radio and
television.[22] There were also the minutes of a meeting at which the
book *At Your Own Risk* by Ralph Lee Smith was discussed.[23] As it
turned out, the AMA had had a heavy hand in both its contents
and circulation, even as it touted the book as having been "independently written." Copies of this book were circulated to 1,200
libraries in the United States as well as to schools, school counselors, legislators, and the media.[24]

What scary material this was! And it was directed at every
chiropractor in America—no one was exempt. But it finally
offered a plausible explaination for much of what my colleagues
and I had been subjected to in the 1960s, as well for who was
responsible. If this information was true, it spotlighted activities
going on within the heavily guarded walls of the American
Medical Association that the organization would certainly have
an interest in keeping quiet. A furtive but very aggressive effort
to completely destroy the chiropractic profession appeared to
have been organized behind the closed doors of the AMA. This
is the stuff of which scandals are made—incriminating indeed.
One thing became certain in my mind: The chiropractic profession could no longer sit back and tolerate what was happening.

* * *

A copy of *In the Public Interest* fell into the hands of Gerald
Hosier, an attorney specializing in antitrust litigation who was
a junior partner with a large law firm in Chicago. He received
the book from a close friend of his, a chiropractor who had been
his college roommate. Hosier read the book and was increas-

ingly astonished and disturbed by the revelations it contained. He felt that it would be unwise, indeed outright foolish, for chiropractic as a profession to allow a situation such as this to go unchallenged. Its failure to stand up to this could only encourage the AMA to become more aggressive in pursuing its demise. Hosier learned from his chiropractor friend that I had recently written a book on chiropractic that also exposed the malicious lies being spread about the profession, and the two of them felt that I might be the appropriate person to contact regarding the serious implications of the charges so profusely documented in *In the Public Interest.* He asked me what the chiropractic profession was doing in response to the revelation of these documents, and wondered whether or not its legal counsel intended to take action.

Hosier said that if the documents contained in *In the Public Interest* were legitimate—and there was no reason to believe they were not—they clearly revealed the fact that the AMA was violating the federal antitrust laws in its efforts to subdue and destroy chiropractic as a competitor to medicine. However, he explained, the book, and the unauthorized copies of the documents it contained, did not provide the kind of solid proof that could stand up as evidence under critical scrutiny; at best, they could be labeled allegations. To prove that the information was true, the original documents would have to be searched out by someone with the proper authority to publicly expose them. The only way to do this would be to subpoena them from the AMA files by initiating a legal action that would enter them into the public record of a federal court.

* * *

Antitrust is an issue that dates back to the nineteenth century. At that time, ruthless businessmen would lower the prices of their commodities until smaller businesses, unable to compete, would either be bankrupted or driven out of business. This would give the larger company a monopoly, and it could again raise its prices, as it no longer faced competition. Left unchecked, this practice would have destroyed the American economic system.

Recognizing the serious implications of this problem, Senator John Sherman helped to draft the Sherman Antitrust Act of 1890, which declared the formation of monopolies and combinations in restraint of trade (to prevent free competition) to be illegal. This congressional act penalized offenders with heavy fines, providing such huge compensations to the injured parties that even the biggest giants in business and industry were discouraged from being so foolish as to take the chance of risking an antitrust lawsuit. In 1914, Congress passed the Clayton Act, which permitted victims of antitrust violations to sue the violators for damages. The Federal Trade Commission Act, also passed in 1914, established the Federal Trade Commission to enforce the law and further prohibited the use of unfair methods of competition in commerce.

Healthy competition forces businesses to provide the best products and services they can deliver at the best possible prices. Everyone wins. Destroying competition opposes every ethical and economic principle on which American commerce is based. To focus more clearly on the damage this can produce, imagine for a moment that General Motors, Ford, or Chrysler formed a special committee with a noble-sounding name like the "Committee on Automotive Quality," but whose primary mission, boldly stated in written documents, was to contain and ultimately eliminate its competition. Imagine that the corporation then publicly slandered its competitors' products so thoroughly with negative propaganda and lies that consumer confidence in the competitors' cars dropped, and the competitors were forced out of business. Then imagine that documents outlining the plot were released to the government and the media. What would be the reaction? We would probably witness one of the biggest antitrust lawsuits ever filed in the history of the United States, which would literally ruin the guilty automaker.

When I had compiled the material for my book, the evidence had pointed toward the existence of just such a conspiracy. Now it was baldly obvious to me that it was indeed the American Medical Association that was the central source responsible for the massive amounts of antichiropractic propaganda that had been circulating for the past ten years. I was disgusted to think that an organization so widely respected and trusted could be so deceitful and underhanded. As Americans, we expect that most of our freedoms will be protected, whether or not they are expressly listed as constitutional freedoms. We take for granted freedom of choice in religion, politics, business—and indeed in health care. Certainly there is more than one valid approach to health. Dr. Benjamin Rush, a physician and signer of the Declaration of Independence, wrote: "The Constitution of the Republic should make provision for medical freedom as well as religious freedom. To restrict the art of healing to one class of men and deny equal privilege to others will constitute the Bastille of medical science."[25]

And perhaps that was the point we were reaching. The AMA had clearly violated federal antitrust laws when it attempted to eliminate chiropractic as a competitor by spreading negative propaganda and advocating a boycott. It seemed appropriate to me for one of the professional associations for chiropractors to take on the AMA in an antitrust lawsuit. There are two national chiropractic organizations in the United States, the American Chiropractic Association (ACA), and the International Chiropractors Association (ICA). (*See* Appendix III, National Chiropractic Organizations, for further information.) These groups had the muscle to institute legal action and the membership to support it—if only they would endorse such an action. Previously, during the effort to have chiropractic included in coverage under Medicare and Medicaid, I had communicated with one of the attorneys who represented the legal interests of chiropractic at the national level. Now I again wrote letters to him, this time exhorting him to pursue legal action on behalf of chiropractic against the AMA for illegally trying to create a health care monopoly.

The top leadership of the ACA, the larger of the two national organizations, normally turned over on a yearly basis. Because of that, the leaders tended to rely heavily on a man who wore two hats. Harry Rosenfield was both legal counsel and Washington lobbyist for the ACA, and the organization's leaders tended to follow his advice without question. While many members of the ACA insisted that taking legal action against the AMA would be appropriate, Rosenfield was of the opinion that more could be accomplished through dialogue. The consensus among the ACA leadership as a whole was that since the organization retained an expert and paid for his advice on matters such as this, they should listen to him.

The ICA, on the other hand, was represented by an attorney

named James Harrison, who judged that litigation would be appropriate if adequate legal representation could be secured. This would mean finding a law firm with the manpower, expertise, and commitment to stay with what was sure to be a long, hard-fought, and expensive battle. Some members within the ICA strongly opposed litigation, but here, as at the ACA, legal counsel prevailed, and the ICA *provisionally* endorsed, in concept, an antitrust lawsuit against the American Medical Association.

It soon became crystal clear to me, however, that no one within either of the professional organizations was going to take the lead in this battle. Someone else was needed to take the reins to get the process in motion. And a finger seemed to be pointing at me: the ICA's endorsement depended upon someone finding appropriate legal counsel to represent us in the suit, and attorney Gerald Hosier had approached me on the recommendation of his chiropractor friend. As much as I dreaded being in the lead, realizing the time and effort it would take and the notoriety that would follow, I was convinced this cause was of paramount importance if choice in health care was to be an American freedom. In good conscience, I could not walk away now. Unless I decided to pursue it myself, it would never be acted upon.

Ardith agreed that this kind of commitment was the only answer to the dilemma and gave me her full support. And so, putting aside my fears, and resolving that we *would* succeed, I pledged to take on the AMA on behalf of chiropractic.

3

GATHERING THUNDER

Armed with my research, my book, the support of information from the pages of the underground book *In the Public Interest*, and solid advice from antitrust attorney Gerald Hosier, I began touring the United States as a guest speaker at state chiropractic conventions, and also being interviewed on radio and television programs. As I traveled, I was able to take the temperature of my professional colleagues and gauge how much support I could expect to rally for a legal action against the American Medical Association. What I found, though, was that virtually any interest I aroused would shortly be quashed by the attorney for the American Chiropractic Association, Harry Rosenfield.

While visiting the state chiropractic associations as an invited speaker, I found myself faced with a typical scenario: The majority of the chiropractors in attendance would enthusiastically support the idea of taking legal action against the AMA. On occasion, they would even take the issue so far as to pass a resolution, sometimes unanimously, in support of it. After returning home, I would wait for a copy of the resolution to arrive in the mail. When it didn't, I would phone the state association's president, only to be told that the resolution had been withdrawn after further consideration—and after the state officers had conferred with Rosenfield.

I contacted Rosenfield to ask why he was discouraging support for the lawsuit. He told me he believed that suing would be a serious mistake for several reasons. First, he said, the lawsuit would give legislators an excuse for not voting on proposed laws relating to chiropractic care (although in reality, there wasn't even a remote connection between the two). Second, he maintained that chiropractic had historically accomplished more through legislation than through litigation, noting that it was legislation that had given chiropractic licensed status in all fifty states, in spite of medical opposition. Third, he said that in Louisiana, in the one instance in which chiropractors had tried litigation as a vehicle to achieve state licensure, the case had been lost miserably. (This was true, but in the first place, the plaintiff in this case, *England* v. *Louisiana State Board of Medical Examiners,* received such bad legal advice that it was amazing the profession had tried to gain licensure in this way; in the second place, the case had no relevance to the merit of an antitrust lawsuit.) Fourth, Rosenfield argued, the AMA would seek to justify its actions by insisting it was protecting the public against dangerous quackery, and to do this it would parade before the public a battery of extremely prestigious witnesses who would all testify to the dangers of chiropractic health care, thereby adding to the barrage of negative propaganda against the profession.

Fifth, and finally, Rosenfield said that he and the ACA were reluctant to get involved in any legal action against the AMA, arguing that it would undermine any possibility of continuing the dialogue between chiropractors and officials of organized medicine that was currently taking place. If the ACA filed a lawsuit, the AMA would consider it an act of aggression, and it would destroy all dialogue and negotiations between the AMA and the ACA, and it would prompt the AMA to become even more aggressive—it would be like waking a sleeping giant.

I was disappointed by the "don't-make-waves" mentality of my profession, by the lack of assertiveness of our leaders, and by their almost apologetic attitude toward what was happening—all of which, I was convinced, was encouraging the AMA to even greater hostility. What, I asked, could the AMA possibly do to harm chiropractic that it hadn't already tried? I considered it imperative that we finally send a message to the medical organization that we had had enough of their lies, and that we were no longer going to passively bear their deceit, attacks, and illegal activities.

I wrote letters to all of the state chiropractic associations outlining the reasons why I believed litigation was the most reasonable approach, and why it was so urgently needed to stop the AMA's illegal conduct against us. I documented how positive accomplishments within our profession had met with increasing hostility and unfair propaganda from the AMA. I reasoned that chiropractic could never hope to grow and advance if it allowed itself to be put down at every turn.

In addition to contacting the professional associations, I contacted many of the chiropractors in the Chicago area. I realized it would be necessary to start a fundraising committee if an antitrust effort were ever to get off the ground. Most of the doctors were enthusiastically supportive of the idea of a lawsuit against the AMA—until it came time to put their names down on a charter. Then they would get cold feet. Apparently their fear of taking on a power as great as the AMA deterred them from offering any support that went beyond lip service. Soon I realized that I would have to conduct a national search for doctors who would be willing to become involved.

A fear of involvement was also gaining a toehold in my own backyard, although I did not realize it then. Ardith too felt apprehensive about taking on a giant like the AMA. She worried about the level of ruthlessness of the people in the leadership of that organization. And she worried about my safety and that of our three daughters, wondering if the AMA would somehow use its muscle to lash out at us personally, or do something to hurt us. But she kept her anxieties to herself, and never mentioned them to me until the lawsuit was initiated and we had the other plaintiffs and our lawyers on our side.

In May of 1974, I went to Greensboro, North Carolina, to speak on three radio and three television talk shows. My trip was arranged and privately funded by Dr. Collin Haynie, who had read some of my articles calling for support of litigation. He hoped to pave the way for me to address the North Carolina Chiropractic Association, which would hold its spring convention while I was in town. By this time, the AMA propaganda machine was going full throttle. Chiropractic needed to respond assertively to this propaganda and bring the facts into perspective, or else the AMA would be encouraged to be all the more aggressive in its attacks. To me, there was and is a critical difference between assertiveness and aggressiveness. Assertive people respond. Aggressive people react. Assertiveness in communication means taking a bold and confident teaching position, expressing your message and clearing the air of misinformation. Aggressiveness is hostile and combative, disregarding the rights of others in pursuit of its own ends.

Dr. Haynie approached the North Carolina Chiropractic Association's state president, Dr. Curtis Turner, and urged him to include me on the NCCA convention program. The president balked at the idea, saying that I was "too controversial." Once again, the fear of getting out of the comfort zone prevailed. But although I did not speak before the NCCA, I did get a chance to do the media blitz in Greensboro that Dr. Haynie had arranged. In the most effective way I knew how, I fought back and exposed the inaccurate propaganda.

I had seen Collin Haynie when I was a freshman in college. He was an upperclassman, so I had never had the occasion to speak with him then. Nonetheless, he had made an impression. He stood well over six feet tall, and his build reminded me of Li'l Abner from the cartoons. In fact, he was an accomplished bodybuilder, having won the Mr. Chicago, Mr. Illinois, Mr. Miami Beach, and Mr. Junior America bodybuilding titles. Additionally, he was on the team that defeated all the regional colleges and universities and brought the midwestern weight-lifting championship of the United States to the National College of Chiropractic. Prior to his chiropractic education, he had distinguished himself in the U.S. Army Air Force as a pilot of twin-engine B-25 bombers during World War II. He was a brilliant man who had accomplished more in his early years than most do in a lifetime, yet a more down-to-earth and nicer person could not be found anywhere. The latter could also be said of his wife, Audrey.

Collin and Audrey had a magnificent estate built on the rolling hills outside of Greensboro. The landscape was majestic. The estate had its own lake, with points and bays and one of the most picturesque shorelines I have ever seen, all encircled by a pathway. Beautiful weeping willows gently draped the edges of the shoreline. A short distance from the shore was a pecan tree. The lake was well stocked with a variety of huge panfish and largemouth black bass that could reach two feet in length. Vegetation was abundant, and the hillsides were dotted with many pine trees, interspersed with huge and impressive oak and walnut trees. The estate was so large and so private that Collin said even skinny-dipping could be done in total privacy—although he qualified that by saying, with a half-smile and a twinkle in his eye, that he wouldn't recommend that men try this if the fish were biting well that day.

Collin and I strolled along the pathway around the shoreline, and as we talked, I began to realize that there were chiropractors out there who were willing to stand up and risk everything for the sake of the truth. Collin and Audrey Haynie were such people. A more gentle and loving couple I have never known in my life. They were courageous individuals who drew their strength from a much higher power. They felt they had been richly blessed on earth and were bound to give something back. Chief among their blessings was not, as one might have supposed, their beautiful home and professional accomplishments, but Collin's very life. In March of 1960, he told me, he had been stricken with a mysterious illness that rendered him unconscious. He spent seven weeks in the hospital in a coma, undergoing all sorts of tests and treatments—and, unfortunately, reactions to the treatments that made his condition even worse—and doctors still had no idea what was causing the coma or what to do to help him. Finally, in frustration, a neurologist suggested to Audrey that she consult with some of Collin's chiropractic colleagues to see if they had any ideas. One of these colleagues, Dr. Joseph Griffith, suggested a cervical (neck) adjustment. With the permission of the neurologist, and as he and Mrs. Haynie looked on, Dr. Griffith performed the adjustment on Collin in his hospital bed. Amazingly, within two hours, he regained consciousness, and two weeks later, he was discharged from the hospital.

Collin assured me that once I formed the necessary committee to initiate the legal action against the AMA, I could count on him to stand by my side. In that beautiful setting, I enjoyed the beginning not only of a new friendship, but also of a great new alliance. I began to believe that we were destined to succeed, although I knew it would not be easy.

Late that evening, Collin and Audrey hosted a buffet dinner in their beautiful home, inviting as guests several of the chiropractors who had been at the convention. Since I could not attend the convention, Collin said, he decided to bring some of the convention's chiropractor members to me. The feedback I got from chiropractors concerning my appearance on the talk shows was positive, but they were also apprehensive because I was making waves. I used the opportunity to present the facts once again, face to face, and to explain why we needed to organize to become more assertive and take legal action against the AMA. I was convinced that there was no way our profession would ever earn its rightful place in health care if, instead of taking a stand for the good we knew chiropractic was achieving, we remained soft and allowed the vicious attacks of our adversaries to continue. The group still appeared nervous and unsure. This was a whole new experience for them. They were unaccustomed to taking this kind of a bold stand and fighting back. Instead, they had been programmed to take the licks and the punishment, hoping that things would eventually blow over and get better. It sounded to them like a wild-eyed dream to take on a giant like the AMA and win. Our cause was right, and they knew that it was right, but the AMA had both wealth and public support. Even our own leaders continued to be divided about what to do, as our experts—including, once again, Harry Rosenfield—advocated the avoidance of any confrontation.

I continued to speak at various state chiropractic meetings, seeking to enlist other allies in the cause of the suit. My speaking engagements took me to many states, including California, where I had an opportunity to meet with Dr. Michael Pedigo of San Leandro. He was a big fellow, built like a linebacker for the San Francisco 49ers. Pondering the AMA propaganda material, with intense determination reflected in the tightness of his square jaw, and with his knuckles turning white, he said, "We've got to do something about this!" He indicated there was nothing he would love to do more than to take the AMA to court. He assured me that if litigation was feasible, I could depend upon his wholehearted support. There was no mistaking his commitment to stand alongside me to the very end, and I knew that I had found an ally in my struggle.

My travels took me also to the state of South Dakota, where I met Dr. Allen Unruh, one of the most successful chiropractors in the state and the public relations chairman of the South Dakota Chiropractic Association. He was a well-read and very positive individual. He had read much of my material and was absolutely convinced that unless we took legal action against the AMA, our profession would continue to invite hostile attacks that would undermine its progress. He was another very strong supporter who I believed could be relied upon when the time was right. I expected he would become another solid ally and a significant force behind this movement.

In Michigan, my path crossed with that of Dr. Clair O'Dell, a prominent chiropractor who had always been an activist for chiropractic. He was a very unselfish and giving person, as well as extremely enthusiastic and positive in his thinking. He also enjoyed immense professional success. In his many years of practice, he gave generously to philanthropic causes. He was one of the founders of the American Chiropractic Association, and more recently Dr. O'Dell provided funding to help start a new chiropractic college. Dr. O'Dell indicated his willingness to support legal action against the AMA. Not only did he passionately believe that our cause was right, but he was convinced that we could be the ones to make it happen.

Thus I had assembled a list of names of colleagues who were supportive of the idea of a lawsuit. I recognized that this support group was not a typical group of doctors of chiropractic. They were special. And they all were winners. Collin Haynie, Michael Pedigo, Allen Unruh, and Clair O'Dell were extremely successful, each in his own right. Each also had a lot to lose materially if things didn't go well in this undertaking. But not one of them hesitated to do what he believed was right and had to be done. We all got strength from each other.

Now that we had rallied the troops—from North Carolina, California, South Dakota, and Michigan—together we formed the National Chiropractic Antitrust Committee (NCAC). The committee was a nonprofit organization dedicated wholly to the advancement of chiropractic interests and to raising the funds to finance a lawsuit against the AMA. On October 17, 1974, we officially wrote a charter, got the papers in order, and continued to pursue the endorsement of a national chiropractic association so that we would be able to apply for tax-exempt status with the Internal Revenue Service. Our tax-exempt status was approved on March 4, 1975, and at that point we were able to begin collecting funds. According to the charter, officers were to include a chairman, a secretary, a treasurer, and trustees. Clair

O'Dell became chairman; Allen Unruh, a trustee; Collin Haynie, treasurer; and I became secretary. Michael Pedigo served initially as a trustee and later became a cochairman. Dr. William Holmberg of Rock Island, Illinois, served as a fundraiser for the Antitrust Fund Raising Committee (AFRC), an arm of the NCAC. He was later voted in as a trustee as well.

According to its charter, the four primary functions of the NCAC were:

1. To improve the working conditions for chiropractic.
2. To take whatever legal action is necessary to stop the American Medical Association from practicing a restraint of trade against chiropractic, as well as to stop the AMA's unfair, unethical antichiropractic propaganda, which is intended to dissuade public opinion from chiropractic.
3. To work for the professional interests of the entire chiropractic profession as well as the interests of the health care of the public.
4. To work as an autonomous organization, yet to be acutely concerned about serving those state and national chiropractic organizations that have supported this committee.[1]

Massive funds would ultimately be received from people within the profession for the purpose of litigation, but the members of the committee would never, in any way, personally receive any of the money that was gathered. If any funds remained once the task of the NCAC was finished, the committee agreed that the remaining funds could be given to our colleges and research projects in chiropractic.

The Congress of Chiropractic State Associations was scheduled to meet at the Holiday Inn in Rosemont, Illinois, on October 25 and 26, 1975. This congress was primarily intended for the state presidents and the state association lawyers. The state presidents met in different forums to discuss their problems and how to cope with them, so that they could bring information back to their respective states. The attorneys convened in a separate meeting room for similar discussions. The format provided a fine occasion for the state leaders and their lawyers to explore avenues for advancing the cause of chiropractic. With the NCAC officially organized, we hoped that the congress would provide our committee with an opportunity to address both the state association presidents and their lawyers, and ideally to get a resolution passed in favor of support for litigation. We sent a formal appeal to the chairman of the congress, Dr. F. Donnell Hart, requesting the opportunity to address the presidents. Dr. Hart, I knew, was not supportive of the lawsuit. He replied, in a letter dated October 11:

Dear Dr. Wilk:

Thank you for your letter of September 27 and your request to address the Congress of Chiropractic State Associations. After consulting with the Executive Committee, it is their opinion that the full Steering Committee should be apprised of your request, and it will be their final decision whether to allow you to address the presidents assembled in Chicago.

The Steering Committee will meet in Chicago on October 24 and make that final decision. If you would contact me at the hotel some time on the evening of October 24, I will apprise you of the board's decision. I am sorry I cannot give you advance approval at the present time. The committee felt it should be a decision made by the entire Steering Committee.

> Very truly yours,
> F. Donnell Hart, D.C.
> Chairman, Congress of Chiropractic
> State Associations[2]

Disappointed, but not totally discouraged, all of us in the NCAC leadership decided that we should plan our own meeting to run concurrently and attend the congress meeting at our own expense.

After we all arrived at the meeting of the congress, we were informed that due to the heavy agenda, they could not give us any time whatsoever during the meeting—not even five or ten minutes—but that they would give us time on Sunday afternoon after the meeting adjourned. But by that time, the state presidents and any other representatives would have left to go home, and we would be speaking to the hotel's cleanup crew. Under the circumstances, nothing we could do would have had an impact.

We observed the meetings from the sidelines, feeling totally helpless. They could easily have given us ten minutes of time on the agenda. But they had apparently been so prejudiced by the

ACA counsel, Harry Rosenfield, that they were unwilling to listen to the opinions that we now brought from two world-class antitrust specialists. Appalled, we watched as they squandered time in arguments over worthless trivia and foolishness, and we realized that they could in fact have easily afforded us thirty minutes—not just the ten minutes we had requested. I was furious that our entire committee had traveled at personal expense from various points across the country to make a vital presentation, and that now, rejected, we were bound by bureaucratic chains and not permitted to speak. If this was the mentality of this profession, then God help us, because we were in trouble!

Since the congress refused to give us time on the program, and presenting our case after the congress adjourned wasn't an acceptable alternative, we made the desperate decision to crash the meeting of the lawyers, which was going on in another room. I announced to the twenty-two lawyers in attendance at the meeting that we had an antitrust specialist willing to explain the merit of an antitrust action against the AMA. Gerald Hosier had said he would be willing to meet with the state association lawyers in his office after hours and explain to them the basis for a suit. We had arranged for transportation for all of the state association lawyers, and we told them cars would be waiting and available for them at the hotel's front door when their meeting adjourned. Then we held vigil on their meeting so that when it broke up, we could again remind them of the available transportation before they left the conference room.

Their meeting adjourned and we told them again that we had arranged for transportation to take them to our attorney's office. Then they dispersed, and we followed them. As they clustered in small groups in the hotel lounge to chat and drink cocktails, we again offered the waiting transportation. Our invitation was ignored by all, except for one lawyer, the attorney from the Indiana Chiropractic Physicians Association. The others ignored our repeated requests.

Watching all of those lawyers sipping cocktails in the lounge, without displaying the slightest interest in or even idle curiosity about the information we had to offer, was almost more than I could bear. I was near tears with disgust at what I saw. It was bad enough that their conduct was indifferent toward our offerings, but these lawyers were being paid by state associations that had retained them in good faith as their representative counsel, and that had sent them here because they were supposed to advocate for the associations' interests. To me, the lawyers were demonstrating an appalling breach of trust.

That lone attorney from Indiana, who elected on his own to take us up on our offer, met with Gerald Hosier. By the time he returned to the hotel, he was absolutely convinced that we had a sound and valid case. The following day, he shared those thoughts with the other lawyers and tried to convince them to consider supporting a lawsuit against the AMA. He was not successful, but he was so insistent that the group finally compromised, and recommended in their final report that further study be done to determine the merit of litigation.

The report of the lawyers was presented at the closing meeting of the congress on Sunday morning. The congress chairman slowly read the report, which opposed support for our lawsuit, then quickly, and almost inaudibly, read the addendum that the attorney from Indiana had managed to have added, which proposed that the organization "explore the facts and law in relation to initiating of a private or governmental antitrust action against the AMA and submit a written report to the members."[3] Perhaps it was because the chairman did not support the added resolution, or maybe it just happened that way, but apparently no one even heard the new recommendation. We asked several of the delegates who attended if they had heard the added paragraph calling for additional evaluation of the merit of litigation, and not one of them had.

I am usually upbeat about everything I do. I strongly believe that whatever we really set our minds to do, if we totally commit ourselves to the goal and never quit, we will ultimately prevail. One of my favorite sayings is that a winner never quits, and quitters never win. If that old proverb was ever strained, it was on that cold evening in October, after the disastrous Congress of Chiropractic State Associations meeting had adjourned and the presidents had gone home. I was disgusted, outraged, and thoroughly frustrated. It was the lowest point in my entire professional career. I knew that we were right, and that the chairman and the lawyers' group had been wrong, but there was nothing I could do.

Dr. Collin Haynie, who had flown in from North Carolina to be at this meeting, put his arm around me and said, "Chet, don't let this thing get you down. Remember that when the going gets tough, the tough get going." Collin is a gentle giant. The old saying that the bigger they are, the nicer they are, certainly applies to him.

Dr. Mike Pedigo had flown in from California. He added, "We've gone this far and we can't quit now. It is much too important."

Dr. Al Unruh, who had come in from South Dakota for the meeting, added, "We cannot let these setbacks stop us. We must continue onward."

Dr. Clair O'Dell from Michigan agreed. "We must simply recommit ourselves until we win."

Everyone else on our committee seemed undaunted and, if anything, all the more committed to achieving our ultimate objective. Together, we seemed to encourage each other. There was beautiful chemistry among us. We were all completely united in our determination to hang in there at all costs and not let this situation stop us from achieving our ultimate goal.

In retrospect, I do not know what it was that angered me more—the so-called experts representing chiropractic interests who were allowing our profession to be trampled into the gutter, or the AMA for its outrageous lies and fraudulent conduct against chiropractic. The conclusion of the members of the National Chiropractic Antitrust Committee was that we had had enough of both groups. In any case, something had to be done about the blindness and lack of backbone of the leadership in the state chiropractic associations, which was allowing the outrages against our profession to continue. If necessary, we would simply have to deal with our leaders and their so-called experts much more harshly. Up to this point, I felt we had been mild, trying to achieve our purpose with minimal public criticism. Now, in light of the behavior of the state presidents, their attorneys, and all the others in trusted positions of leadership with the national chiropractic associations, I prepared to become more and more publicly critical, until these individuals either behaved with more professional integrity or were humiliated into taking appropriate action. Either this strategy would help us ultimately to prevail, or we would be seen as outrageous fanatics. In either case, the facts were on our side. The other members of the NCAC agreed with me that the war had begun.

I went home that evening feeling great about the unity and commitment expressed by the committee. This was the ultimate test, I felt; if we could keep going despite this setback, then we could overcome any adversity. Out of every negative and grave situation, some good seems to come, and the good here, I felt, was that our committee was proving itself to be indestructible and undauntable. In reality, our strength and success came not from winning, but from rising up after failing and recommitting ourselves to our goal.

* * *

The next morning, a large envelope addressed to me unexpectedly arrived at my office. Inside were about fifty clippings from newspapers across the United States, all on the subject of the AMA's disinformation campaign regarding chiropractic. They were articles written about an informant from within the hierarchy of the AMA who called himself Sore Throat. By this time, I was already somewhat familiar with this alias because it had appeared in the press. Some unknown individual (using a name that called to mind the informant Deep Throat of the Watergate scandal) had sent packages containing copies of internal AMA memos to reporters, congressmen, and government agencies regarding, among other things, the covert and overt activities of the AMA toward chiropractic. He had also sent copies to Ralph Nader of Public Citizen Health Research Group and to major newspapers. Some of the documents he revealed had already been exposed in *In the Public Interest,* but the sudden appearance of Sore Throat attracted media attention in a way the book had not, no doubt because of the mystery he created and the fact that the tips he gave reporters usually proved to be worth pursuing. The AMA was in a dither over who might be sending this damaging intraoffice information to the press and to members of the government, and even hired a detective agency to uncover his identity.

Attached to the clippings was a note to me, which stated that the sender of this material was none other than Sore Throat himself, and that if I wished to speak to him, I should be prepared to accept a collect call from a "Dr. Throat."

Imagine my excitement! Just yesterday I had hit what seemed

to be the bottom, and suddenly this package arrived, from the same Sore Throat who was already causing quite a stir in the United States Congress and in the newspapers—not to mention within the AMA hierarchy. And I would be able to speak to him myself!

About two days later, I received the collect call from Dr. Throat. His voice was rather soft and gentle, if slightly raspy, and I will never forget it. He identified himself only as a medical doctor who was bothered by what he had seen in the internal files of the AMA. He said he knew all about me because the AMA had a dossier on me, and my name kept coming up as someone who would like to take the AMA to court. He indicated that he had called the ACA lobbyist on different occasions, but that Harry Rosenfield had not seemed cooperative or willing to support any legal action; therefore, Sore Throat had given up on him for the most part. Then he contacted me, hoping he could provide some assistance that would help to bring about a law-suit. He said he would like to do what he could to help rectify the unjust things that he had seen happening, and he asked how he could help.

This voice from an unknown distance stirred tremendous interest in me. He was saying the same things I had been saying for the past couple of years, but my words had seemed to fall on deaf ears. It occurred to me that this mysterious voice might finally be the one to arouse the chiropractic profession to action. I gave Sore Throat the names of several top officers of the national chiropractic associations so that he could communicate directly with them; then I alerted several of these chiropractors, who indicated they would gladly accept his collect calls. I never knew how to reach Sore Throat myself, but had to rely on his making collect calls to me. He appeared to make his calls from pay telephones in the Washington, DC, area, and he never called from the same phone twice.

Soon after this, Sore Throat wrote an open letter to me in support of a lawsuit against the American Medical Association. He intended it to be shared with as many people in the chiro-practic profession as possible. The letter was succinct and pow-erfully stated. It clarified the AMA's motivations, detailed the AMA's misconduct, advocated an antitrust lawsuit, and stressed the need for urgency. I immediately passed it along for publication in *The Journal of Clinical Chiropractic*. I also arranged for Sore Throat to speak at a seminar for chiropractors given by Dr. James Parker that was to be held in Dallas, Texas. Dr. Parker was regarded as a "practice-builder" within the profession, an entrepreneur who helped chiropractors build their practices and make them more successful. His seminars had initially been developed to teach chiropractors the business end of chiropractic, an aspect not covered in the curricula of the chiropractic colleges, but later these meetings were expanded to provide a broader exposure to all aspects of chiropractic, including the medical, motivational, and business sides. I regarded Dr. Parker as someone who could show chiropractors how to survive in the very hostile and negative climate created by the AMA propaganda machine. He was incredibly successful in his seminars, and always drew large crowds. Even Ronald Reagan attended one of them during his 1980 presidential campaign.

It was arranged that Sore Throat would speak via telephone to those gathered at the seminar, with his voice amplified by a sound system connected to the telephone receiver. Dr. Parker arranged to use a device to distort Sore Throat's voice so that it could not be recognized. This exposure generated more interest than I had been able to accomplish in almost two years of traveling and public speaking. Perhaps 2,000 chiropractors— some of them in the highest ranks of chiropractic leadership— and their staffs attended the seminar where Sore Throat was scheduled to speak.

Finally, the doctors were beginning to listen. With newspapers throughout the country carrying the articles prompted by Sore Throat, and the stir about a potential congressional inquiry into antitrust action against the AMA, chiropractors were not only belatedly realizing that what the NCAC was saying had substance, but also that they had been sold a bad bill of goods by their own ACA lobbyist in Washington. They were recognizing that not only antitrust specialists but even congressional attorneys were concurring with what the NCAC had been saying for the past year. And now, with their eyes opening for the first time, they listened.

When Sore Throat finished speaking, Dr. Parker addressed the chiropractors and stated, "I want you to understand I am not supporting it. You can either support it or not. I have no policy on it." For Dr. Parker to take that position at his own seminar killed any hope of broad economic support. Had he instead appealed for funds at that moment, the result would have been very different.

I heard from Sore Throat only one more time following that meeting. He telephoned me to inquire how the doctors had responded to his speech. I reported that significant interest had finally been generated, but that it did not bring the kind of economic response we had hoped for. He sounded both frustrated and discouraged when he replied, "Well, I've done everything I can for you. From this point you're on your own." I suspect he considered it to be a waste of time to try to help people who apparently did not have the good sense to try to help themselves by standing up and fighting with the ammunition they'd been given.

I never heard from Sore Throat again, and I never found out his true identity. Years later, I encountered a person who claimed to be Sore Throat, but his voice was definitely not the one that had so mysteriously first contacted me in late 1975.

At about this time, the American Medical Association apparently began to suspect that a lawsuit would soon be filed, and that the activities of its Committee on Quackery might be a serious liability. Shortly before the leaked AMA documents began to appear in the press in the summer of 1975, and eleven years after it began its work, the AMA's Committee on Quackery was dissolved and the Department of Investigation was dismantled. At that time, the department described itself as a success, even though during its existence chiropractic had achieved licensing in all fifty states, as well as limited coverage by Medicare. The primary reason cited by the AMA for discontinuing the office and its committee was financial.

*   *   *

Following the meeting of the Congress of Chiropractic State Associations, it was the NCAC that complied with the resolution adopted by the congress attorneys calling for additional study of the feasibility of litigation. We retained one of the nation's foremost attorneys specializing in antitrust, Professor Paul Slater from Northwestern University School of Law, to conduct a scholarly and objective in-depth study of the antitrust issue. This man was above reproach as far as any personal interest in the case was concerned, since he would not litigate the case. Neither did he have any chiropractic interests.

During this same period, the correspondence between Harry Rosenfield, the ACA legal counsel in Washington, and me became extremely heated and candid. He continued to oppose litigation against the AMA, while I continued to plead for it. The state associations became more and more confused, as Harry and I kept colliding head on with each other, neither of us relenting. With the legal advice and encouragement of Gerald Hosier, I was prepared to persist at all costs, believing this was the right thing to do.

Rosenfield never did, in fact, object to the lawsuit on the basis of whether or not there were possible legal grounds for it; he merely maintained that such a suit was unwise from a political point of view. He proposed instead leaving it to the national and state legislatures to fight the fight for chiropractic. He justified his position by stating that without litigation, chiropractic had been licensed in all fifty states; insurance-equality legislation had been passed guaranteeing the right to use any state-licensed form of health care; chiropractic had been approved for coverage under state and federal workmen's compensation plans, Medicare, and Medicaid; and the U.S. Department of Education had officially granted the Council on Chiropractic Education the responsibility for accrediting chiropractic colleges and ensuring the quality of chiropractic education. Rosenfield maintained that litigation would be counterproductive for chiropractic in the issue of national health insurance, which he saw as the most pressing issue at that time, and might turn legislators against us when they considered laws affecting chiropractic care. He further denigrated the suit by depicting it as an intramural fight between medicine and chiropractic—in other words, merely a squabble among the components of the healing arts, not unlike what happens within professions.

By the end of 1975, my communications with Harry Rosenfield became so intense they might even have been called a dogfight. Certain influential chiropractic leaders, who had originally suggested that the timing of the lawsuit might not have been the best, were now urging Rosenfield, in light of new evidence such as the information from Sore Throat, to reconsider the proposed suit. Rosenfield stubbornly refused to budge. He rejected all requests to wait for the findings of attorney Paul Slater's antitrust study, and continued to denounce the suit as lacking merit.

With my new determination to be more publicly critical of Rosenfield and the ACA leadership, and in the spirit of giving fair notice, I sent a letter to the ACA attorney advising him that the NCAC was not going to tolerate the current direction of the ACA on this matter, and that we were thenceforth planning to deal with them more harshly. "Harry, I am hereby submitting you and the American Chiropractic Association notice to be more careful in the future with statements relative to our antitrust movement," I wrote. "Your record on the antitrust matter is a sad one, and the documents speak for themselves. If necessary, and if in the interest of chiropractic we are in a situation where we must take very harsh measures against you or the ACA, please be advised that we will."[4] I hoped that my threat to make public the soft policies of the ACA leadership regarding the issue of an antitrust suit would create enough discomfort for them to come to their senses.

The leaders and legal counsel of the International Chiropractors Association (ICA), the smaller of the national professional organizations, were more willing to listen to the advice of legal experts regarding the need for an antitrust action against the AMA. Further encouraged by their own association lawyer, James Harrison, who recognized the merit of litigation, the association offered conditional endorsement for the lawsuit, subject to their attorney's final approval. This in turn depended on the NCAC being able to find legal counsel with the ability, experience, and staff to handle the job. This was no small order.

Finally, Paul Slater completed his study for the NCAC. He concluded that chiropractors did indeed have a very solid basis for taking the AMA to court for violation of the antitrust laws. He very clearly expressed his opinion for appropriate action when he told me: "Those people at the AMA had to be incredibly stupid and arrogant to have put into writing their plans for the containment and elimination of chiropractic, but that stupidity can only be surpassed by [that of] the chiropractors if they do nothing about it."[5] Slater became the third antitrust specialist who agreed that this case had substantial merit.

With the results of Slater's study, and encouraged by the

conditional endorsement of the ICA, the members of the National Chiropractic Antitrust Committee began searching in earnest for an attorney to represent chiropractic's interests in the antitrust lawsuit against the AMA. Gerald Hosier had already proved to be an exceptionally bright and capable attorney. As an antitrust specialist associated with a patent-antitrust law firm, he was certainly qualified, and he had an excellent record of success in the cases he had represented. However, he was only a junior partner in his law firm. To take on a giant like the AMA and some of its allies would be beyond his resources and experience; regardless of how brilliant he was, he would be buried by the size of the massive task this promised to be. We needed a senior partner, antitrust expert, and trial lawyer who had the solid support of a large law firm and who was not only seasoned by experience but also had ample staff to provide the clerical, paralegal, and research assistance that would be needed.

Attorney George McAndrews came into the picture at this point. He had in fact already conducted his own fairly extensive study of the antitrust issue, both because of personal and family-related interests and because it was his own area of legal expertise. He too felt that we had a cause for action. However, despite the fact that he was an expert in patent and antitrust law and senior partner in a large law firm, he did not want to take on the case himself. His brother, Dr. Jerome (Jerry) McAndrews, was the executive director of the International Chiropractors Association and one of the most respected administrative leaders in the chiropractic profession. George did not want, and did not feel it would be appropriate, to have any appearance of nepotism shadowing the selection of our counsel.

I was introduced to George by his brother, Jerry. George is about five years younger than I, and a graduate of Notre Dame University. He is a tall man, athletically built and well proportioned. In high school, he had played in state championship basketball, and had distinguished himself in setting Iowa state records in the discus. He still had the look of an athlete. My first impression of him was that he was very much in charge of any situation, and he was very articulate.

We met in George's office in the Loop to discuss securing a firm to take the case against the AMA. George felt we had a basis for the case if we kept it on the narrow basis of antitrust only, rather than including questions of slander or libel. He agreed to search on behalf of the NCAC for another antitrust specialist affiliated with a large law firm who would be willing to take the case. He contacted eight different Chicago law firms and followed up on all recommendations. Unfortunately, every firm he contacted that might have been able to handle a case of this scope declined, and all for the same reason: They were representing drug manufacturers, medical societies, or other medically oriented interests, and they simply did not want to accept a chiropractic case that might be construed as a conflict of interest, thereby running the risk of losing their current clients. The other candidate firms were so small—in one case, a single-attorney law firm—that they were actually less able to handle the case than Gerald Hosier would have been. Finally, after some time had passed and all other possibilities for law firms had been exhausted, the NCAC implored George to argue the case himself.

This case was the last thing he needed. The truth was that we would be a financial liability to whomever accepted the case. Although we anticipated getting the support of a national chiropractic organization, we could not provide assurances that adequate funds would come in to support the tremendous costs of litigation.

In the early months of 1976, George McAndrews finally accepted the case on its own terms. He felt that he had no choice—that if he did not, it would never get off the ground. The lawsuit still needed the endorsement of at least one of the national professional organizations. Without that endorsement, it was doomed before it began; there would be no chance of rallying the economic support from chiropractors that we needed to fund the case. The ACA attorney continued to discourage chiropractic support for legal action at every opportunity. The ICA's endorsement was provisional, depending on their approval of our attorney. George could find no one else with the talent and the staff to represent us appropriately. So if the case were ever to be brought, he would have to do it himself.

* * *

The principles inherent in the suit mattered to George in a personal way. He came from a chiropractic family. In fact, his family tree included an impressive list of twenty-seven chiropractors. His brother was a chiropractor and a leader in the ICA; a sister and several other members of his extended family also were chiropractors. His late father too had been a Doctor of Chiropractic—the first chiropractor in that total number of twenty-seven.

In 1928, George's father was dying. His medical doctor's diagnosis was severe asthma. George's father was six feet four inches tall but by then weighed only about 160 pounds. In order to be able to breathe, he frequently had to hang by his knees from a bar that was braced in a doorway. Epinephrine (Adrenalin) was the drug used in those days to help such patients, and it was usually administered every four hours, but George's father had to take it every fifteen minutes. One day, George's mother heard of a new kind of doctor in their Wisconsin community—a chiropractor. She convinced her husband to try chiropractic. After only three visits to the chiropractor, he never had another attack (*see* Chiropractic as a Treatment for Asthma, page 76). Soon afterward, he himself became a chiropractor.

While his physical affliction ended, George's father suffered a different kind of agony—encountering scorn and prejudice because of his profession. He felt great empathy for the suffering of other people, and he brought relief to many who had been in pain for years. But he also saw his beloved profession ignored and denigrated, sometimes by people who could have benefitted from his care. On more than one occasion he found himself having to make house calls at two or three o'clock in the morning—not because it was an emergency or because he was that busy, but because a patient did not want his neighbors to know he was receiving a chiropractic adjustment. Sometimes the denigration could get personal; he was even rejected for membership in a local country club because he happened to be a chiropractor. Years of rejection and frustration over what he knew was a terrible wrong led to deep depression, which ultimately contributed to his hospitalization and a premature death.

So for George, our case on behalf of chiropractic had a strong personal meaning. He only had to recall his father's experience. If he had any thoughts of declining to take it, he said, he had a mental image of his father kicking the lid off his burial vault in outrage to say to him, "I put you through college and law school. Do you mean to tell me you're not going to use your education

Chiropractic as a Treatment for Asthma

Chiropractic is primarily identified as helpful for neuromusculoskeletal problems. However, there is some anecdotal evidence that it may be helpful for other types of ailments as well, probably because chiropractic treatment acts on the spine, and the nervous system plays a role in virtually all bodily processes.

Asthma is one condition for which a full research trial of chiropractic intervention is merited. Anecdotes and personal and clinical experience have shown results, but the scientific community puts little stock in these, so clinical double-blind studies are needed. Such experiments are very expensive, however. Recently, a pilot study entitled "The Role of Chiropractic Treatment in Chronic Childhood Asthma" was initiated. The projected cost of this study is $85,094, and it is being funded by the American Chiropractic Association, through the Foundation for Chiropractic Education and Research, in memory of George McAndrews' father, who was cured of what had been diagnosed as life-threatening asthma by chiropractic treatment.

and ability to come to the rescue of my profession now, when they need it and you have the opportunity?" It seemed to George that he was being led to right a serious wrong in this nation, to begin to open a window on the ignorance, bigotry, and discrimination that for decades had imprisoned his father and others like him—not to mention the countless people who never were enlightened about a type of health care that could have eased their suffering or even saved their lives. A man of deep compassion as well as understanding for our cause, George McAndrews came to realize he had no choice but to take the case himself.

The ICA had given us its support of the suit contingent upon final approval of our selection of legal counsel. With George on the case, the organization's endorsement was a foregone conclusion. George was a senior partner in a major law firm that represented some of the largest Fortune 500 clients. More than that, he was simply a brilliant lawyer. He had graduated from Notre Dame University with a degree, with honors, in mechanical engineering. He had been selected as Engineer of the Year in 1959. At law school, also at Notre Dame, he had been Editor in Chief of the Law Review. He had been honored with a clerkship for a judge on the United States Court of Appeals for the Seventh Circuit (including Illinois, Wisconsin, and Indiana). The ICA immediately endorsed our choice of attorney, and declared its support of the lawsuit on March 14, 1976. We were off and running.

* * *

We had to work quickly to prepare the lawsuit because we suspected, as Sore Throat had suggested, that the AMA was purging its files and shredding incriminating documents. Still, it would take another seven months before plaintiffs with verifiable injury from the illegal boycott would make known their willingness to file suit.

With the NCAC's tax-exempt status, we were free to raise funds for litigation. On March 22, 1976, The ICA sent out a mass mailing to chiropractors throughout the country notifying them of the organization's endorsement of the suit and urging all the chiropractors in America to offer their financial support.

The response was overwhelming. Funds poured into the NCAC from all across the United States and Canada. This was something the AMA had not expected. They had never considered that a suit might be filed without the support of the ACA, and the ACA's opposition to litigation had encouraged them to continue their hostilities toward chiropractic. Now they knew they were destined for a battle.

Many individual chiropractors donated thousands of dollars. There are many chiropractors who are financially very well established and who enjoy impressive state-of-the-art clinics, palatial homes, luxury cars, large incomes, and other tangible symbols of success. In spite of that, however, they still experience the pain of rejection and prejudice. No price tag can be put on respectability, and the propagandists had tried long and hard to strip this from them. One colleague expressed to me how it pained him to deal with condemnation from people ignorant of the healing value of his art. He told me about a time when his daughter had come home from the school playground, sobbing after being taunted by children who were ridiculing her father's profession. She threw her arms around her father's neck and cried, "Daddy, you're not a quack, are you?" Tears welled up in this man's eyes as he remembered the incident. This doctor and others not unlike him were now facing a moment when they could use the fruits of their success to fight for recognition as the true healers they are, and they reached out to grab it.

As members of the chiropractic profession began to realize that a sincere effort was being launched to file a lawsuit against the AMA, the NCAC was contacted by doctors who had suffered personally from the boycott on chiropractic by the medical monopoly. Four of these people stepped forward to ask if they could become named plaintiffs in the case. Dr. Patricia Arthur was one such person. In the small town of Estes Park, Colorado, she had applied to the local hospital for the privilege of sending patients to them for radiological services. They agreed to this arrangement. On the basis of that assurance, she invested all of her available money into preparing and opening her new chiropractic office. On the day her practice opened, she received calls for appointments from many new patients. Several of the patients were sent to the local hospital for their initial x-rays. To Dr. Arthur's dismay, every one of her patients was denied access to the much-needed x-rays. Only then was she told that the code of ethics of the AMA, which was shared by the American College of Radiology, denied the hospital the freedom to cooperate with her. Thus, she had signed a lease, prepared an office, and bought furniture, treatment tables, and all of the other necessities for conducting her practice, but she was denied access to radiological services. Then, Dr. Arthur said, while she was appealing the denial by eight medical physicians on the hospital staff, her patients had to travel sixty miles through the mountains to another chiropractor's office for necessary x-rays. The appeal process resulted only in her profession being defamed by the AMA propaganda machine, and the resulting news coverage upset her efforts to build a practice in the small community. Her decision to abandon her practice and leave the state of Colorado was illustrative of what the AMA was able to do to hundreds, if not thousands, of other licensed professionals. She felt crushed by what had been done to her. When I first spoke to Dr. Arthur, she was outraged, nearly to the point of tears, and she was fighting mad—but she didn't have the money to take on the medical establishment by herself. This became her opportunity to fight back. She asked to become a plaintiff in the suit against the AMA, and we offered to assist her.

Another chiropractor who came forward as a plaintiff was Dr. James Bryden of Sedalia, Missouri. He was a man of small build whose appearance reminded me somewhat of Don Knotts, who played the role of Barney Fife in the *Mayberry* television series. That is where the resemblance ended, however. This man was intense, tough, and not to be intimidated; he was very much in control of what he wanted to accomplish.

Dr. Bryden was concerned about certain patients who had come to him with pain behind the sternum. Such pain can be a sign of heart trouble that requires medical treatment. Whenever he had a patient who he suspected might have a heart condition, Dr. Bryden would run an electrocardiogram (EKG) test to help determine whether the pain was a result of a joint dysfunction or a sign of a heart problem. Then he would send the EKG tapes to the local medical cardiologist, Dr. Jerome Block, who would read and interpret the tapes and then provide a written report on his findings. In this manner they worked cooperatively for a time, until the rumor began circulating in the Sedalia hospital that a local medical doctor was "dealing with chiropractors." A surgeon in Sedalia decided to do his own research to discover who that doctor might be. He had his secretary call some chiropractors in town and say that she needed a chiropractor for her elderly mother, who was moving in with her. She would claim that her mother also had a heart ailment, and would wonder aloud who the chiropractor would utilize in case her mother experienced heart problems. When Dr. Block's name came up and it was established that he was cooperating with chiropractors, he was summoned before the Bothwell Memorial Hospital Ethics Committee.

Although Dr. Block had done nothing involving chiropractors inside the hospital's walls, the ethics committee threatened to revoke his hospital privileges. He was advised that the hospital could not allow any of its member doctors to associate with chiropractors, and that if he continued to cooperate with any chiropractors, they would consider this behavior unethical and he would be suspended from the hospital medical staff. Dr. Block humbly accepted the admonishment. Realizing that continuing to cooperate openly with Dr. Bryden would be professional suicide, but also realizing that Dr. Bryden was acting properly in consulting on possible cardiac cases, Dr. Block followed his own sense of obligation and agreed to continue to cooperate with Dr. Bryden, but covertly. This meant giving reports by telephone rather than putting anything in writing. As a result of this experience, Dr. Bryden was justifiably angry at the conduct of the hospital, and demanded that justice be done. He was more than eager to take on the medical establishment.

Dr. Michael Pedigo and I decided that we also would become plaintiffs. The damages we had suffered were typical of those of thousands of chiropractors—injuries perhaps less pointed, but that nevertheless took place on a daily basis as a result of the illegal boycott, such as the denial of hospital cooperation.

I maintain a small convenience office in my home in the Chicago suburb of Park Ridge, Illinois, for emergencies and for the sake of neighbors who occasionally receive adjustments there. However, my home office has no x-ray equipment. On one occasion, I sent a patient to the nearby hospital for x-rays, having in advance received a letter from the radiology unit indicating they would accept my patients for diagnostic x-rays. When my patient arrived there, she was refused the service. The incident was unpleasant for us both, as well as a personal embarrassment for me, since her daughter was a close friend and classmate of my own daughter. Ultimately, the woman had to make the long trip into the city to go to my Chicago office for the x-rays. Not only does this illustrate the effect of the boycott, but it was also a breach of contract for which the hospital could be sued. The person who wrote me the letter saying the hospital would perform x-rays for me clearly didn't realize when he signed it that a code of ethics mandated by the AMA prohibited cooperation with chiropractic.

Finally, one other chiropractor, Dr. Steven Lumsden, expressed his desire to become a plaintiff. This made a total of five chiropractor-plaintiffs. In the end, however, Dr. Lumsden experienced a personal tragedy not long after the suit was filed, and because of this, he had to withdraw as a plaintiff in the case. He had always been strongly supportive of the case and his heart was with our cause; he still regrets that he was not able to stay with it until the end. Ultimately, however, only four plaintiffs were able to see the case through.

The antitrust lawsuit was filed on Columbus Day, October 12, 1976. This suit would subsequently be referred to in documents as *Wilk* et al. v. *American Medical Association* et al. In addition to the American Medical Association, fourteen other defendants were named. The list of defendants included the American Hospital Association; the American College of Surgeons; the American College of Physicians; the Joint Commission on Accreditation of Hospitals; the American College of Radiology; the American Academy of Orthopaedic Surgeons; the American Osteopathic Association; the American Academy of Physical Medicine and Rehabilitation; the Illinois State Medical Society; the Chicago Medical Society; and four individuals: H. Doyl Taylor; Joseph A. Sabatier, M.D.; H. Thomas Ballantine, M.D.; and James H. Sammons, M.D. Taylor, Sabatier, and Ballantine were influential members of the AMA's Committee on Quackery, the special committee created for the sole purpose of eliminating chiropractic in the United States. Sammons was an executive vice president of the AMA.

It was apparent that we were literally taking on the entire medical establishment. The organizations and individuals named as defendants had established themselves as the authorities on health care, and we were challenging their conduct. Not only did they enjoy the trust of the American people, but they seemed to have unlimited funds with which to fight for their interests. We knew we were right, but without the commitment and financial support of our profession, we had no hope of success. We could not do it alone; even with the help of our colleages and our lawyers, it was a David-and-Goliath type of undertaking. But we felt that if truth and honesty had any meaning, we would have to prevail in the end. We were poised and ready.

4

THE CLOUDS ROLL IN

At the time the lawsuit was filed, the American Chiropractic Association continued to oppose the action. Not only had they adopted a resolution in opposition to the suit, but they also advised the membership of their organization not to support the litigation in any way. The association leaders maintained that as long as the ACA was retaining an expert to advise them on legal matters, including the position to take on this issue, its members ought to listen to that counsel. This expert, of course, was Harry Rosenfield, the ACA's legal counsel and Washington lobbyist.

The leadership of the International Chiropractors Association, on the other hand, endorsed the lawsuit, now that their attorney had given his final approval to our choice of lawyer. If the ACA attorney had supported the suit, I had no doubt that the organization would have gotten behind it immediately.

It should be mentioned that the ICA membership did not unanimously support the litigation. Some within the ICA hierarchy actively opposed the suit, ridiculing it and calling it the "Joe and Jerry Show," after ICA president Joseph (Joe) Mazzarelli and executive director Jerome (Jerry) McAndrews (who was also the brother of our attorney, George McAndrews). Interestingly, Drs. McAndrews and Mazzarelli, together with a group of other chiropractors, later switched their membership to the ACA.

Meanwhile, George McAndrews stopped working for the National Chiropractic Antitrust Committee. His role changed when he started representing the plaintiffs; as an ethical matter, he could work for either the NCAC or the plaintiffs, but not both.

Now he devoted his efforts to preparing the case for the plaintiffs. There was no guarantee that enough money would ultimately be raised to pursue the case to a successful conclusion, and this presented a problem. It takes funds to pay clerical and support staff. So George limited his use of other staff until the trial was upon us. He had already agreed to write off any portion of his own fee and related expenses that exceeded the funds we succeeded in collecting, so this case had the potential to be an incredible financial liability for him.

In the four years between the day we filed the suit and the day we went to court, there were depositions, interrogatories, document searches, and travel. The legal profession refers to this period as *discovery*. The object of the discovery phase is to enable each side to obtain information and materials to help them determine the facts and prepare for the presentation of the case. During this time, our attorney was given the right to search the files of the AMA for evidence to substantiate our claims. He put in long hours at AMA headquarters, copying all kinds of documents that would eventually be entered as evidence into the court record during the trial. George compiled volumes of evidence to support our case. Because he was doing most of the preliminary work himself, George ended up traveling to thirty-four states to take depositions of a total of 165 witnesses. A deposition is a process in which a witness is questioned under oath by lawyers for both sides, and the testimony is recorded by a court reporter. It aids in the discovery process, and the testimony may later be introduced as evidence during the trial.

Chiropractors from all across the United States cooperated as well, coming forward with relevant documents supporting our allegation of antitrust violations. In total, over a million documents were ultimately amassed. This represented a compilation of more documents than had ever been processed by George's law firm in any single action. For the sake of security, the law firm kept all the documents in a locked room that had a steel door with a special tamper-proof lock. Had the keys to this door ever been lost, it could have been opened only with a blowtorch.

At times it seemed quiet where we were, but as plaintiffs we had an acute sense that for the time being, we were in the eye of the storm. The defendants literally ganged up on George, sometimes with depositions to be taken on the East Coast on one day and others on the West Coast, with different lawyers, a day or two later. In spite of it all, he remained in good humor—smiling, joking, and simply taking it in his stride. These were especially hectic and stressful days for him. He stood alone under a tremendous amount of pressure, and I insisted that he come to my office for chiropractic adjustments. The treatments relaxed him. He remarked that whenever he received an adjustment, he would sleep like a baby that night.

It is not an easy task to prove in a court of law that an organization is deliberately attempting to destroy its competition. As plaintiffs in this antitrust litigation, we were faced with the burden of proof. Three things had to be proved:

1. That there had been *intent* on the part of the defendants to eliminate competition.
2. That the defendants had *implemented* that intent with bold action.
3. That the defendants had been *successful* in their elimination program.

Based on the accumulation of documents compiled from various sources, our case was constructed on the following five-point basis:

1. That the AMA had attempted to contain and eliminate chiropractic.
2. That the AMA had cooperated and worked with the other named defendants to boycott chiropractic and totally isolate chiropractors from other members of the health care community.
3. That the AMA had attempted to prejudice government studies on chiropractic.
4. That the AMA had operated through private organizations to bar chiropractors from professional access to public facilities such as hospitals and universities.
5. That the AMA had wrongly influenced insurance companies to deny chiropractic coverage to patients.

From AMA headquarters, documents from meetings of the association's board of trustees were secured by our attorney. These spelled out in black and white how the AMA had formed a special committee expressly to plan, and be held accountable for, the elimination of the chiropractic profession. This committee had outlined step by step, in writing, how this was going to be done.[1] Finally, and again in writing, the AMA Committee on Quackery had reported to the board how successful they considered themselves to be in their containment and elimination program.[2] We were able to amass considerable evidence from the files of the defendants themselves to support all three of the necessary aspects of our charge of antitrust violation, and this convinced us more than ever that our case was sound. But the American Medical Association still had to be found guilty in a court of law.

The internal documents revealing the AMA's cleverly orchestrated antichiropractic campaign, with its boldly stated intent to contain and eliminate chiropractic, were a major support in the building of our argument. How could they deny their motives when they were so clearly stated in writing? The Committee on Quackery's master plan for the demise of chiropractic had been developed by an attorney who originally represented the Iowa Medical Society, Robert B. Throckmorton. He was concerned about the rapid growth of chiropractic in Iowa and the possible threat it posed to the practices of physicians and surgeons. Speaking before the regional North Central Medical Conference in Minneapolis on November 11, 1962, he had addressed what he called the menace of chiropractic, labeled the profession a cult, and called for a "positive program of containment."[3] He urged a national crusade against chiropractic. The outline of his plan included a broad list of proposals designed to destroy chiropractic both from within—through encouraging "chiropractic disunity" and "stifling chiropractic schools"—and from without, by encouraging ethical complaints against chiropractors, prohibiting chiropractic care in hospitals, and opposing the inclusion of coverage for chiropractic in health insurance and workers' compensation programs, Medicare, and labor union health plans. Further, he cautioned that this should be done covertly: "Any action undertaken by the medical profession should be . . . behind the scenes whenever possible." And he gave one absolute directive for medical doctors: "Never give professional recognition to chiropractors."[4]

After his impassioned speech in Minneapolis, Throckmorton

was hired as the general counsel for the AMA, and as they say, the rest was history.

Cooperating with the AMA in its antichiropractic campaign were some opinionated characters who claimed to be protecting consumers, but who in fact were spreading outrageously distorted information. Many of these individuals spoke at state medical conventions to build opposition to chiropractic. They were, in reality, opportunists who capitalized on the occasion to spread antichiropractic propaganda. They did this in a way specifically designed to create prejudice among unsuspecting doctors, who attended these conventions looking for new information to bring back to their own practices, and who tended to believe what they heard at these gatherings.

Dr. Joseph A. Sabatier, Jr., was one such individual. He was a physician from Louisiana who served as chairman of the AMA's Committee on Quackery. According to notes taken at a 1973 meeting of the Michigan State Medical Society, at which he was a guest speaker, Sabatier felt that "rabid dogs and chiropractors fit into about the same category. . . . chiropractors were nice people but . . . they killed people. . . it is very important to point out to members of the medical profession that it is considered nothing less than totally unethical to refer patients to a chiropractor for any purpose whatever."[5] Five days after that meeting, the Michigan State Medical Society adopted a resolution declaring it unethical for M.D.s to refer patients to doctors of chiropractic for any reason.[6]

The key participant in the AMA's closed-door operation was H. Doyl Taylor, an attorney, who was hired in January 1965 as director of the American Medical Association's Department of Investigation. He also was made secretary of the Committee on Quackery. This put at the disposal of the committee the vast facilities of the Department of Investigation, with its extensive resources—money, personnel, and access to all kinds of information—as well as intricate networks for planning and organization. Taylor helped to write the explicit antichiropractic policy statement that called chiropractic an "unscientific cult whose practitioners lack the necessary training and background to diagnose and treat human disease" and "a hazard to rational health care" (see page 46).[7] This statement was based on Principle 3 of the AMA's "Principles of Medical Ethics," adopted in

1957, which prohibited medical physicians from associating professionally with unscientific practitioners:

> A physician should practice a method of healing founded on a scientific basis; and he should not voluntarily associate with anyone who violates this principle.[8]

Not until after our lawsuit was filed did the AMA change its official statements condemning all chiropractors (*see* The AMA Reverses Itself . . . Or Does It? on page 89).

In 1964, the AMA's Department of Investigation successfully influenced the National Educational Association (NEA) to adopt a resolution stating that "consumer education" materials prepared by the AMA would be distributed in the public schools.[9] As a result, the NEA circulated thousands of pieces of antichiropractic propaganda literature to educators and school guidance counselors. This move undoubtedly had an impact on the career choices of countless young men and women who might otherwise have considered pursuing chiropractic as a profession— not to mention biasing a massive number of young public school students against chiropractic care.

During the discovery phase before the trial, a scandalous document was revealed regarding the report on the 1968 need and cost study by the U.S. Department of Health, Education, and Welfare (HEW). This was the study ordered by the Congress as it considered the issue of including chiropractic among the professional services eligible for coverage under Medicare (see page 35). A letter dated March 11, 1968, from Dr. Samuel Sherman to H. Doyl Taylor advised Taylor of the outcome of the study even though the study was not scheduled to begin until August of 1968, *five months later*.[10] This letter proved that the report's findings were rigged and the study was a sham. This tainted report had been a major victory for the Committee on Quackery in their defamation campaign against chiropractic. Some individual members of the committees involved in the study were disgusted enough by what they had seen to make their documents available to us as evidence. For instance, Walter Wardwell, a professor of sociology at the University of Connecticut, responded to a subpoena by producing a box of documents from the time he served on the Expert Review Panel for Chiropractic,

The AMA Reverses Itself . . . Or Does It?

Our lawsuit against the American Medical Association was filed on October 12, 1976. By that time, the organization's policy statements condemning chiropractic had stood as guidelines for several years and were the basis of the illegal boycott of the profession. When the lawsuit was filed, the AMA suspended distribution of its antichiropractic policy. Apparently hoping to head off the lawsuit, the AMA's House of Delegates, which oversees medical policy issues for the association, adopted a new policy statement on chiropractic, known as Report UU.[1] This document stated that some things chiropractors did were not without therapeutic value, but it stopped short of saying that these services were based on scientific standards.

In 1980, the AMA revised its "Principles of Medical Ethics," deleting Principle 3, which had banned consultation with "unscientific" practitioners.[2] In theory, this appeared to end the AMA boycott of chiropractic. In effect, however, the attitudes of the leadership of organized medicine did not change. It is important to note that even as of December 1980, when the trial began, the AMA was continuing to mail outdated antichiropractic literature in response to requests for information on chiropractic.[3]

Naturopathy, and Naprapathy, and he later testified at the trial. Other committee members, however, had destroyed their files and other evidence. (The sad postscript is that even after the HEW study was exposed as a sham, the AMA continued to refer to it as an independent government study that rejected chiropractic.)[11]

During discovery, it was learned that Taylor had also worked behind the scenes at meetings to help author the 1969 policy statement on health care for the Health Insurance Association of America (HIAA), which had advocated the exclusion of coverage for "manipulative services and subluxations for the purpose of removing nerve interference."[12] (See page 38.) This wording was aimed directly at chiropractic without mentioning it by name, since chiropractic is the only therapy that uses this approach to health care. When chiropractors protested the wording, the HIAA said only that it could not control how its statements were interpreted. The policy statement seriously undermined insurance company relations with chiropractic.

That was not the full extent of Taylor's influence as a writer of propaganda for groups outside the AMA. The article condemning chiropractic that had appeared in *Senior Citizens News* in 1969 had been widely distributed (and reprints of it financed) by the AMA, which claimed that the article represented an independent viewpoint from outside medicine (see page 36). In fact, however, it had been formulated and edited by Taylor.[13] This article had been a major propaganda blow against chiropractic and was full of false information. It had been circulated by the AMA to legislators in Washington, particularly those on the House Ways and Means Committee, who were then deciding the question of whether to include coverage for chiropractic in the Medicare program.

That Taylor figured prominently in the entire operation to eliminate chiropractic was evidenced by the fact that his name seemed to appear everywhere on internal documents relating to chiropractic—to a greater extent even than we had expected it to. While some of the material was openly attributed to him by name, Taylor also had ghostwritten a substantial amount of published material over the years that had cast a shadow on the integrity of chiropractic. Some of his writings were uncovered during the discovery phase; other information did not surface until the trial was actually underway. The various propaganda pieces included the NEA consumer education resolution against chiropractic, the HIAA policy statement, the dishonest and now discredited HEW Report, and the *Senior Citizens News* article. He was also involved with the 1969 book entitled *At Your Own Risk: the Case Against Chiropractic* (see page 42).

The AMA had promoted *At Your Own Risk* as having been independently written by an author named Ralph Lee Smith. Nowhere between its covers did the name of the American Medical Association appear. But, in fact, the AMA had financed the publication and dissemination of the book. Hundreds of thousands of copies were printed, and copies were sent to every library, school, legislator, and anyone else who might have had some influence on the subject. This widely circulated book violently attacked chiropractic and had a very damaging impact on public confidence in the profession. The book contained countless statements of contrived misinformation that could be disproved. But the negative message about chiropractic continued to be circulated throughout America by means of this book, and its misinformation continued to be quoted as fact. The book was an effective and powerful tool for the AMA. There is no question that, for his part, Doyl Taylor did a magnificent job both as a writer and as a choreographer of injury to the chiropractic profession for the benefit of his bosses at the AMA. He was indeed the master of the negative propaganda we had seen.

* * *

In the discovery phase, the defendants' lawyers required that each of the five plaintiffs submit names of the patients they had treated over a period of months, so that the defendants could request the court's permission to open our patients' files. I gave them my complete mailing list in response to their demand. Any patient who came forward claiming to have been unhappy with his or her doctor or treatment, for whatever reason, was a candidate to become a prime witness for the defense.

In the meantime, my own legwork on behalf of our cause continued. Ever hopeful of getting the American Chiropractic Association to reverse its position opposing the lawsuit, I made an appeal before a meeting of the ACA in Houston in June of 1977, about seven months after the suit was filed. Initially, my prepared speech had a very mild tone, but the NCAC felt that the time had come for the message to be stronger and tougher, to awaken the ACA delegates from their complacency. No longer did we have anything to gain by being likable or by stroking the egos of the delegates, and so the text was rewritten to tell it like it was. I quoted the 1963 decision of the AMA Board of Trustees on its mission to contain and eliminate chiropractic, noting that they had been trying to turn chiropractic into a pseudoprofession, and make it impossible for chiropractors to improve their education, ethics, or professional competence—

the very things, I reminded them, that were the primary objectives of the ACA. As members of the organization, I said, they had a duty to honor these objectives. (For the full text of the speech, *see* One Last Attempt to Rally National Chiropractic Support, page 93.)

When I finished speaking, the faces of the audience were grim. Not one person was smiling; no one stood up to agree with me, or spoke up to say that it was time to stand up and be counted. In fact, as the delegates gathered in small clusters within the larger room, the expressions on their faces, and the tone of the mumbling in the room, reflected pain and anger—and it appeared that most of their anger was directed at me. No one moved toward me to say that he or she agreed with what I had said.

Finally, one of the delegates did approach me. Quite disgusted, he said, "You insult them, you knock them down, you kick them in the ass, and then you ask for support. You are dead. They will never support your cause. You are talking to a bunch of prima donnas. You can't talk to them that way and expect to get their support. You have just buried any hope you may have had for support."

"If that is true," I responded, "then it will be too bad for the delegates and the ACA, because we will pursue and win the suit without them. This organization will end up being on the outside looking in. They will have cut off their nose to spite their face."

Through the years, I had often observed that chiropractors vented their anger toward each other with more zeal than they did toward those outside their circle who would seek to destroy them. I witnessed this again in their attitude toward me at the ACA delegates' meeting. It reminded me of the image of two bear cubs tied in a sack. When they cannot escape from their confinement, they start fighting each other, but they could so easily be free if they just worked together to tear open the bag.

George McAndrews believed that in spite of the immediate reaction of the ACA delegates, given time my speech would have a positive impact. While they were initially infuriated by it, they would have to go home and think about what had been presented. It would gnaw at them until they would finally be ready to accept the truth—then they would be able to realize just how vitally important it was for them to step forward and lend

One Last Attempt to Rally National Chiropractic Support

After our lawsuit was filed, I decided to make yet another attempt to persuade the American Chiropractic Association (ACA) to join our cause, by means of a speech delivered to a June 15, 1977, meeting of the ACA. My speech began with an expression of appreciation to the ACA for allowing me to address the delegates, and the comment that I had been uncharacteristically quiet for the past months because I was now one of five individual chiropractor-plaintiffs engaged in an antitrust suit in U.S. District Court for the Northern District of Illinois. I briefly identified the defendants as the American Medical Association, the Joint Commission on Accreditation of Hospitals, the American Osteopathic Association, eight other medical groups, and four individuals. "Three of the individuals," I said, "are from the AMA's so-called Committee on Quackery, or what you all know to be the committee created to eliminate chiropractic in the United States." I then began the main portion of my address:

> *This evening I stand before you as an ACA member, and as a chiropractor who finds a glaring contradiction between the stated objectives of the ACA and its activities in the past years.*
>
> *On page eleven of the July 1976 State of the Art publication of the ACA, it states, and I quote: "A primary objective of the ACA is to establish and maintain the standards of education, ethics, and professional competency necessary or desirable to meet the requirements of the profession and the expectation of society."*
>
> *I believe that we can all agree that this is a noble objective, well suited to an organization such as the ACA. I will be making reference to that objective from time to time, and ask that you keep it clear in your mind.*
>
> *Now I'm going to read an objective taken from a memorandum from the Committee on Quackery of the AMA dated January 4, 1971. "Since the AMA Board of Trustees' decision at its meeting November 2–3, 1963, to establish a Committee on Quackery, your Committee has considered its prime mission to be, first, the containment of chiropractic, and ultimately, the elimination of chiropractic."*

Think about that, ladies and gentlemen—a private committee created by a private group to eliminate our profession, notwith-standing that the law in all fifty states endorses our right to exist as professionals and to serve our patients.

Coincidentally, in the same year, 1971, the AMA had published another edition of its Judicial Council Opinions and Reports. That publication continued an attempt to strangle chiropractic by iso-lating it from all contact with other health care professionals, health care institutions, and institutions designed to pay for health care in the United States, such as insurance carriers and state and federal health care compensation programs. It was designed to lower chiropractic into the gutter of pseudoprofession, and it was intended to make it impossible for chiropractors to improve their lot with either improved education, ethics, or professional compe-tency—the primary stated goals of the ACA.

Painful as it is, let me remind you of the gutter treatment accorded chiropractic in the infamous boycott disguised, in part, as an ethical mandate by the American Medical Association and its related groups. Now listen, and listen good.

Page 15, paragraph 8 of the 1971 edition [of the AMA's Judicial Council Opinions and Reports] says: "It is the position of the medical profession that chiropractic is an unscientific cult whose practitioners lack the necessary training and background to diag-nose and treat human disease. Chiropractic constitutes a hazard to rational health care in the United States because of the substan-dard and unscientific education of its practitioners and their rigid adherence to an irrational unscientific approach to disease causa-tion." Paragraph 5 of the same page says: "The physician who maintains professional relations with cult practitioners would seem to exhibit a lack of faith in the correctness and efficacy of scientific medicine and to admit that there is merit in the methods of the cult practitioners." Paragraph 6 of the same page goes on to say, "The principles of medical ethics proscribe all voluntary professional association between doctors of medicine and sectarian or cult practitioners. The giving of a medical paper by a doctor of medicine before a group of cult practitioners by invitation would be voluntary professional association contrary to the principles of medical ethics."

I continued by reading from another section of the same 1971 publication, which related to podiatrists, then commented:

I might add that it seems that chiropractors are used as a bench-mark for worthlessness. . . [It] says that the practice of podiatry is not a cult practice "as is chiropractic. . . ."

Again, I ask you to keep in mind the primary objectives of the ACA in the field of education, ethics, and professional competency, and some of the unarguable facts that have directly flowed from the foregoing attempt to isolate and eliminate chiropractic:

1. *Regarding improving education, we have taken heroic strides to establish and maintain high standards of education, in spite of the fact that certain highly qualified teachers could not teach in our schools without fear of reprisals by the AMA and those over whom it wields control. And this was so whether the educators were skilled in x-ray technology, diagnosis, pathology, physiology, or any of the other scientific disciplines necessary for the education of a chiropractor. The stigma of [being branded as] "unethical" or the threatened loss of hospital privileges of an M.D. is a terrible price to pay for consorting with a chiropractor.*

2. *Also regarding education, we have upgraded our standards of education with superhuman effort, in spite of the fact that our adversaries have willfully done everything within their power to prevent it. They have actually attempted to keep colleges and universities from freely transferring and accepting credits with chiropractic colleges. That's right! Pressures have been brought to [bear to] prevent state and private colleges from instituting cooperative preprofessional college programs with chiropractic professional colleges. This is just another example of tactics employed by the brilliant strategists of the AMA—keep them from being educated, and then damn them for being ignorant.*

3. *Regarding ethics, I ask you, who is it that demonstrates ethical shortcomings when a chiropractor, with the welfare of the patient in mind, refers a medical problem to a medical doctor, knowing that the medical doctor must, in turn, propagandize the patient into believing that the chiropractor is a cultist? When that same medical doctor sees a chiropractic problem, he is forbidden to refer the patient back to a chiropractor. When a chiropractor seeks the assistance of a hospital's facilities or personnel, he is frozen out by the boycott—and the patient be damned!!*

4. *Regarding professional competence and education: In situ-*
   ations where chiropractors in the field have sought to upgrade
   and enhance their knowledge and professional competency
   through continuing education programs, our adversaries
   have made it unethical for knowledgeable health care profes-
   sionals to participate in our programs, or to allow chiroprac-
   tors to attend continuing education programs sponsored by
   those groups, subject to the pressure of the AMA and its
   allies.

On this point, I would like to quote exhibit P from the complaint
in our lawsuit. Exhibit P is a letter from the Chief of Neurosurgery
at the University of California Medical Center, Dr. Phillip R.
Weinstein, and is addressed to the American College of Chiropractic Orthopedists. The letter is dated March 21, 1975, and it says:
"Dr. Ernest Bates and I regret to inform you as per our recent
telephone conversation that we will be unable to lecture at the
forthcoming meeting of the American College of Chiropractic
Orthopedists. I sincerely regret that stipulations in the judicial
council rulings of the American Medical Association, section 3,
paragraph 4, prevent us from participating. Please accept our
sincerest apologies for this late cancellation due to circumstances
beyond our control. We were unsure that delivering medical
lectures to your group was prohibited."
    Again, I refer you to the ACA's stated preoccupation with the
establishment and maintenance of standards of education, ethics,
and professional competency, and I submit to you that it is
absolute folly for the ACA to speak in these noble terms and aims
while treating casually the jackboot of our adversaries buried in
the back of our profession's neck attempting to drive our education, ethics, and professional competency into the gutter!!
    On October 12, 1976, I and four other chiropractors, who have
taken the position that we will not voluntarily stay in the gutter
and who have decided to take the risks inherent in challenging the
irrational and damnable activities of the AMA and its allies, filed
an action against the defendants that I have previously named.
    We had then and we have now the moral and enthusiastic
support of most of the chiropractic profession. Noticeably lacking,
however, was the moral or enthusiastic support of the American
Chiropractic Association. And this is all the more puzzling, because this organization lists as its prime objective the establishment and maintenance of standards of education, ethics, and

professional competency. Are these words merely hollow plati-
tudes of the ACA? Is it possible that views far narrower than the
broad horizons of the goals of chiropractic dictated the attitude of
the ACA? Is the ACA truly determined to establish and maintain
standards of education, ethics, and professional competency for
chiropractic? If so, then pray tell how it can do it without first
doing battle with the illegal and far reaching boycott blanketing
our entire profession.

The battle is not a selfish one. It is joined on behalf of our
patients as well as ourselves. We do battle to right a grievous
wrong to ourselves as chiropractors and, in the ACA's own words,
"to meet the requirements of the profession and the expectations
of society."

On February 9, 1977, the Chicago Tribune in a front-page,
column-one article entitled "Chiropractic: It's Sneered At No
Longer" gave major emphasis to the lawsuit. On February 20,
1977, the Chicago Sun-Times in an article entitled "Chiropractors
Boom Ahead?" made the blanket statement—and I quote—"The
AMA, bitter foe of chiropractic, has pulled in its horns, stung by
an antitrust suit by chiropractors."

Finally, and within the last few months, the AMA has issued
a new [edition of its] Judicial Council Opinions and Reports,
and—listen to this, and listen well—the words "chiropractic" and
"chiropractors" do not appear in it at all. On pages 13 and 14,
however, under the provision entitled Interprofessional Relations,
appears the following: "A physician may refer a patient for diag-
nostic or therapeutic services to another physician, a limited
practitioner, or any other provider of health care services permit-
ted by law to furnish such services, whenever he believes that this
may benefit the patient." It also says, "He may, as well, choose to
accept or decline patients sent to him by licensed, limited practi-
tioners." And it also says, "Physicians are free to engage in any
teaching permitted by law for which they are qualified."

Furthermore, I notice in the AMA News [sic] that the Joint
Commission on Accreditation of Hospitals, a named defendant in
the lawsuit, is planning on amending some of its accreditation
standards involving areas that are strangely and remarkably (but
with tongue in cheek I don't say coincidentally) related to matters
discussed in our complaint.

We are not so blind as to believe that mere window-dressing by
the AMA and its allies has changed these organizations' goal of
eliminating chiropractic. I leave it to the historians and to reasonable

*men to acknowledge the dancing-on-hot-coals response to our adver-
saries to the just claim of me and my four coplaintiffs and our cry for
freedom for ourselves and our patients. I believe that reasonable men
will feel compelled to see that the jackboot that has lain so heavily and
so long on our profession's neck is starting to slip. I suggest it will be
lifted altogether only when our adversaries see that we five plaintiffs
are uttering a cry for professional freedom and dignity that is echoed
by chiropractors across the land.*

*I don't ask for money. I do ask you to treat seriously and
realistically the ACA's objectives of establishing and maintaining
standards of education, ethics, and professional competency. I ask
that you join your voices with those of other state and national
chiropractic organizations and individual chiropractors in en-
dorsing our efforts in the lawsuit now being conducted in Chicago.*

*The boycott curtain has been parted, as demonstrated by the
new words of the AMA Judicial Council, and through this parting
the light of potential rational, interprofessional cooperation has
appeared, and with it can come benefits to society.*

*Together we share a common goal and purpose—the betterment
of the general health of the American people. By helping chiropractors to establish and maintain high standards of education, ethics,
and professional competency, that purpose or end is brought closer
to reality.*

*I submit that the artificial barriers created by our adversaries
must and should be removed with the full and enthusiastic support
of the ACA. The burning question in my mind is: Will it be done
with the enthusiastic support of the ACA . . . or will it be done in
spite of the ACA?*

*Your lack of endorsement to date is a burden that chiropractic
can ill afford. It can only give aid and comfort to the AMA and its
allies as they frantically attempt to modify their irrational policies
as the day of accounting draws nearer.*

*Share with me for a moment, if you will, a vision of the reaction
of the powers that be in the AMA, in view of the activities and
actions that have recently taken place and that I have outlined here,
as their informants deliver to them the news that the ACA has
elected to endorse the activities of the five chiropractors in the
antitrust lawsuit. On the other hand, imagine their relief and
contentment at the ACA's failure to take a decisive stand.*

*Ladies and gentlemen, I ask that you put substance and credibility
into your pledge to establish and maintain the standards of education,
ethics, and professional competency necessary or desirable to meet*

the requirements of the profession and the expectation of society of which you expound. I ask that you be big enough to correct a prior mistake or oversight. I ask that you endorse the actions of the five plaintiffs who have proclaimed to the AMA and those associated with it that we intend to demand our rights and our patients' rights, as recognized by the law of the land, notwithstanding the illegal actions of any private group.

I might say that the obvious slippage of the jackboot and the apparent confusion and uncertainty of its wearer makes my neck feel a bit better and makes each day a little brighter for chiropractic. Now, won't you please help remove it altogether?

Thank you for your time and attention. I trust you will bear with me and understand when I say that I have no further comment on the lawsuit. Again, thank you, and good night!

their support to the cause. He felt that they needed that jolt to come to grips with the realities of the situation.

Needless to say, however, the ACA did not drop its resolution opposing the lawsuit. During the next year, positive developments that occurred with the suit made it increasingly clear that the lawsuit was making progress. When that happened, the ACA changed its stance so that instead of opposing the suit, the organization took no position on it. In effect, the ACA deemed the action unworthy of any policy position at all. This was far less than we had hoped for, and I considered it just one more insult to our cause.

Eventually, in the face of increasing pressure from its membership, the ACA hired a law firm of its own to evaluate the feasibility of an antitrust lawsuit. Antitrust suits are indigenous to major cities like New York or Chicago; there are more antitrust lawsuits filed in a city like Chicago in one day than are filed in some of the smaller states in a full year. But where did the ACA ultimately find a law firm to do its feasibility study? In Utah! However, that firm did advise the ACA that the case had merit. Finally, three years after our suit was filed, the ACA adopted a position of support for the lawsuit, but that endorsement included no financial commitment, and the ACA continued to withhold any pledge of financial support. With the endorsement of the ACA, the organization's legal counsel, Harry Rosenfield, also belatedly went on record in support of the lawsuit and urged chiropractors to support it as well.

* * *

The attorneys for the defendants, in gathering their own evidence, scheduled times for taking depositions of the plaintiffs. They took their initial deposition of me on Tuesday, February 21, 1978, sixteen months after the lawsuit had been filed. That morning was a typical cold, gray wintry day in Chicago. I arrived at attorney George McAndrews' office for a last-minute briefing, then we walked to the office of Perry Fuller, the attorney for the American Academy of Orthopaedic Surgeons. There, fourteen lawyers (including George) and I gathered in a conference room around a large table.

I stood to be placed under oath. The first examining lawyer was Max Wildman, chief attorney for the American Medical Association. His initial questions concerned my background—when and why I got into chiropractic. He noted that I had quit optometry school and wanted to know why. Other questions sought to elicit my basic philosophy on health care, information such as when I graduated from college, and what my experience in the military medical facility had been like. He also wanted to know what kind of examinations I did in the office, what kind of diagnostic equipment I had, and how I treated patients. All in all, it was a fair fact-finding mission designed to help them understand something about the person they would have to face in court. Of course, if they had found anything along the way that would damage my credibility, I'm sure they would have been very receptive to that. It was their assignment to destroy my case, after all.

After probing my background and philosophies, the questioning moved to an evaluation of my patients' history cards—the questions I asked in taking a patient history and what kinds of ailments made up most of my practice. Then Wildman asked, "Have you ever been prevented from rendering whatever services you felt appropriate within the concept of chiropractic as you know and practice it as a result of not being able to associate yourself professionally with a medical doctor?"[14]

After a moment of thought, I told him that the lack of cooperation between chiropractors and medical doctors presented me with a damned-if-I-do-and-damned-if-I-don't type of dilemma. I had the option of sending a patient to a hospital or an M.D., in which case I would risk losing him; or I could choose not to refer him to an M.D. and risk the possibility that the patient might be harmed if he needed medical care. This meant that if I had a patient who needed both the chemical and/or surgical approach of orthodox medicine *and* the structural manipulative approach of chiropractic, I was simply unable to function as effectively and efficiently as I should be able to, in the best interests of the patient.

"Let's take a hypothetical situation," I said. "A person sustains an automobile accident. He is taken into a hospital. That does not preclude the need for chiropractic care. He may need comprehensive x-ray. He may need a surgeon to suture the wound. He may need psychological counseling for the psychological trauma he sustained. He may need physiotherapy. But he may also need chiropractic care and proper, rational interprofessional utilization of all of these in proper perspective. And if I send him to the hospital, I must forsake him chiropractically. If I keep him chiropractically, I must forsake him medically. And I am faced with this damnable situation of being, as I said, damned if I do and damned if I don't. And I realized that I must do everything in my power to break this barrier in the interest of my patients."

Wildman queried, "What do you do when you are faced with that dilemma, as you described it?"

"I get frustrated. I get angry."

"Do you send him to the doctor?" he asked.

"I filed the lawsuit. That's what I did."

Wildman rephrased his question: "What do you do about the patient? Do you send him to the doctor or to the hospital, or don't you?"

Sadly, I replied, "I forsake them sometimes chiropractically."

Wildman persisted, "By that, you mean you send them to the medical doctor?"

I explained, "I send them to the medical doctor, where they may need chiropractic as well, and [having done that] I am unable to give them this chiropractic care."[15]

The last lawyer to question me was the attorney for the American Osteopathic Association, John Duczynski. His questioning was very brief. "To your knowledge and in your opinion," he asked, "is there any condition of ill-being or well-being in a human being in which chiropractic care is contraindicated?"

"I would be remiss in my obligation if I said no to that," I replied, going on to explain that I believed medications might be inappropriate for some structurally related ailments that would respond better to structural type of treatment—and that to keep administering high-powered medications might not only be inappropriate, but might even cause harm in the form of a drug reaction, some other illness, or possibly even nerve atrophy.

Duczynski asked me, "Is there any condition under which chiropractic care is contraindicated?"

My response was, "I thought I answered it, and I would say yes, as medicine is contraindicated, and every profession has conditions which are contraindicated."[16]

Then Duczynski asked me if I had ever had a patient I felt I could not provide care for, to which I responded that indeed I had. And with that, the taking of my first deposition concluded.

A second round of depositions was held seventeen months later, beginning at 8:00 A.M. on Friday, September 19, 1980. Again, I met George McAndrews in his office, and we walked this time to the law firm of Wildman, Harrold, Allen & Dixon, located on the twenty-ninth floor of One IBM Plaza. Like the first meeting, this meeting also started on time, and I stood to be placed under oath to give my testimony. Little else about this encounter was like the previous occasion, however. Immediately it became quite confrontational in tone. We were less than two minutes into the deposition before the lawyers of the opposing sides began to get testy with one another. This meeting and the taking of my deposition took place over two days.

This time, another attorney for the AMA, a man named Doug Carlson, was brought in to question me. With him were eight other attorneys, representing eight of the other defendants. Each of them would have the opportunity to ask me questions.

In response to a last-minute directive from George, I had provided the names of three patients I felt would provide a good overall picture of the kinds of results chiropractic is able to achieve, particularly with patients who failed to get good results with orthodox medicine. The attorneys set about attempting to characterize these patients as ringers, carefully hand-picked by George to create a case against medicine. Such was not the case. The truth was, George had had nothing to do with the selection; these patients had been chosen by me from my own list of active patients.

The first patient they questioned me about was Mary S., a fifty-four-year-old woman who had only recently become a patient of mine.

Carlson was the first to question me. "Dr. Wilk, is [Mrs. S.] a patient of yours?"

"Yes, she is," I affirmed.

"Were you aware before this morning that your lawyer, Mr. McAndrews, has designated in court papers which he filed [Mrs. S.] as a potential witness in this matter?"

"Yes, I have."

"Were you involved in any way," Carlson went on, "in picking [Mrs. S.] from among your many patients?"

"Yes, I was."

"What was the extent of your participation, please?" he asked.

Without hesitation, I explained as frankly as I could. "I was advised that I needed very quickly three patients, and so I went into my office and very quickly selected three people, called them, asked them if they would be willing to be witnesses. They accepted."

Carlson asked his next question deliberately. "You looked through many records, is that correct? Hundreds?" It was apparently his intention to make it appear as though I had gone through an exhaustive list of patients with the intention of picking the three that would support our case.

I answered, "'Many' is relative; not really. I went more or less through active patients."

Carlson asked, "Well, did you go to the file and just close your eyes and pick three?"

I shook my head slightly. "No. I selected three people with histories I thought would be of interest to you."

Carlson raised his eyebrows. "Well, I thought Mr. McAndrews asked you to pick the three and not us, Dr. Wilk. Didn't you think they would be of interest to him?"

I smiled to myself. "I selected three people which I thought would be of interest to the court, [to] everybody concerned."

Carlson knew that I had been giving seminars to chiropractors on how to go to the media with our message and communicate it effectively and accurately. His next remark reflected that, and was the first of several times my seminars would be referred to during the giving of this deposition. He admonished, "Dr. Wilk, this is not a talk show."

My attorney interjected, "Hold it. That is an insult, and you will not do that. He answered your question, and that is all you are entitled to. The preambles can stay out of it."

Carlson defended himself, "Mr. McAndrews, I mean no insult."

"You intended an insult," George insisted. "You so represented it. There is no place in this for that, Mr. Carlson. It isn't a talk show, he answered your question. He is under oath. That is all you are entitled to. Now, ask the question without the preambles."

Then Carlson admonished George, "It is much too early in the morning to be heated here."

George didn't give an inch. "Stop the snide remarks and the sarcasm. He answered the question. He is under oath."

Carlson said, "I suggest to you, and Dr. Wilk, to you, I did not mean it as an insult. I know you have participated in numerous programs, question and answer sessions. All I am suggesting is that this is a different context."

George replied, "He knows it. He just stood and took an oath. He does not do that on a talk show."

Carlson asked, "My question was, didn't you think that the patients that you picked from your files would be of interest to your lawyer?"

I answered the question more fully this time. "I felt it was of interest to the court, to you, to the attorney, to everybody concerned, to provide a more accurate expression of why we are all here. I am sure you are interested in truth as much as I am. I am not being evasive. I am trying to be factual and tell it like it is. I believe I cannot be more accurate than simply saying these x-rays [Mary S.'s x-rays were submitted as evidence] are a good example of what the court would be interested in, and would give a more accurate expression of why we are all here in the first place."[17]

The truth was that these attorneys were less than happy with the selection of this patient as an example. I was even asked whether she was a relative or family friend. She had a history of unsuccessful medical treatments that had been ongoing since she was twenty-three years old. Mary had chronic low back pain that extended down into her legs. She had had her veins stripped, thinking it might correct the problem, but without results; she had tried all kinds of medical care, but nothing had ever helped her; and she had experienced virtually continuous pain until she came to my office. Moreover, she had come only at the urging of her husband, and was openly negative about the possibility that my treatments might help her. That in part was what made her an excellent witness for our side; she was a classic victim of the adverse propaganda against chiropractic, and she had for a long time stubbornly refused to give chiropractic a chance because of it. She did not believe in chiropractic care, but her husband and her friends urged her to try it, and finally she gave in. Such patients are the last ones who would be susceptible to psychosomatic suggestion, which was one of the things the medical propagandists would have had everyone believe was responsible for chiropractic's success in relieving symptoms. The other explanation most commonly offered by the medical establishment is that diseases just happen to "run their course," creating the impression that chiropractic has helped—but after thirty-one years, it was most unlikely that this could be the case. Finally, the attorneys tried to suggest that this woman might have been helped by medical care she received during the same period of time, rather than by the care she received from me. However, I was in fact the only doctor treating her at that time. I knew this because she had told me so. She said that she had taken all kinds of medications for years and nothing helped, and as a result she had given up on medicine and resigned herself to a life of pain. When Mary consulted me, it was without any expectation that I could help her, so she was genuinely surprised by the prompt improvement in her symptoms. During my cross-examination by the defendants' attorneys I commented on her results:

> I am sure you have seen the record—she says this is the first time in 31 years she is totally free from pain. I saw her the other day. I believe I saw her yesterday. She says she has never felt so good since she was 23 years of age, 31 years. This I might add was done in a matter of a few visits.[18]

The questioning continued and at times even became insulting. At one point, the AMA attorney asked, "Why did [Mrs. S.]

have to come back to you in two days and give you $17?" This question was clearly out of line. Patients come for their health, of course—not to give me money! Angrily, I responded, "I object to the innuendo, the $17. . . . I object to the tone. . . . You are a professional man. I wish you would try to conduct yourself in a professional manner rather than trying to insult me with a $17 innuendo. It indicates I am trying to run a monetary—"

George interrupted, "Why did you have to come here and charge your client for it?"

Coolly, Carlson replied, "Dr. Wilk sued my client."

George lost his patience. "That is nonsense. Get on with it."[19]

The rest of the questioning dealt primarily with the two other patients whose histories I had submitted. One was a man who for five months had suffered from headaches and vertigo, and had even been hospitalized for these problems, receiving extensive medical therapy without results. After chiropractic adjustments, he got good relief from the headaches. The third patient had spent ten days at Loyola University Medical Center for sacroiliac (extreme lower back) and leg pains, without results. He responded well to chiropractic treatments.

These three patients provided a fair representation of typical chiropractic patients. They also served to contradict the defendants' claim that chiropractic was worthless, which they offered as justification for their plan to eliminate the profession.

On the following Monday, September 22, the deposition continued. The lawyers asked a variety of questions as to how the several plaintiffs had become involved in the lawsuit. Many of the questions concerned my having formed a speaker's communication program for chiropractors and advocated going on radio and television with the many positive accomplishments of chiropractic. There were questions regarding Sore Throat as well.

Perry Fuller, the attorney for the American Academy of Orthopaedic Surgeons, also questioned me briefly. He represented clients who had more to lose than the average M.D., since chiropractors and orthopedic surgeons treat many of the same types of ailments. Fuller dwelled on the psychosomatic aspects of health care, subtly implying that patients who are helped by chiropractic are more psychosomatically influenced than they are helped physically.

The Illinois State Medical Society (ISMS) was represented by attorney Logan Johnston. His approach was more defensive. He took the position that the ISMS was not a part of the conspiracy, but was more of an innocent bystander. For the most part, he tried everything he could to distance his client from the boycott. His questioning was brief, and his line of questions specifically referred to what I had seen the ISMS do that would suggest it was part of the conspiracy.

Although it was not one of the major, more aggressive offenders in the boycott, the ISMS knew of it, was involved in it, and cooperated with the conspirators. For example, an M.D. named William M. Lees, Chairman of the ISMS Board of Trustees, who was seeking the office of president within the ISMS, was advised that if he wanted to make a name for himself, he should write an article for the *Illinois Medical Journal* and get his name out before the membership in that way. An article was supplied to him and he took the credit for authoring it, although he did not actually write any of it. He was not even sure of its accuracy.[20] This article was an attack on chiropractic. The statements it contained were so outrageous that Dr. Lees could never have been able to substantiate the material, but it was published in the *Illnois Medical Journal,* and it surely did prejudice many M.D.s against chiropractic.[21] George had deposed Dr. Lees and found that not only did he not know whether the material was accurate, he appeared to have little recollection of its content.

Shortly after that article came out, I had, in fact, called Dr. Lees on the phone and proposed having a debate with him on the radio over the content of the article. Johnston asked me about that.

"Who was the first person at the Illinois State Medical society you contacted about the article?"

"Dr. Lees."

"Did you do so by phone?"

"Yes."

"Tell me as best you can recall what you said and what he did."

"In essence," I explained, "I indicated to him that I thought the article was totally deceiving, that it was totally inaccurate, and that it reflected no intellectual or academic honesty, and that I would challenge him to a debate which I had prearranged. His response to that was to the effect, in essence, that he would not debate me. I asked him if he wanted some factual information on chiropractic. He insisted that he did not want any additional help or information from me. It was short. He just had no interest in dialogue with me whatsoever."[22]

* * *

In the final days of pretrial preparation, an atmosphere of intensity was achieved in George McAndrews' office that is still difficult for me to describe. Even to this day, my adrenaline flows as I remember the level of activity and the magnitude of what was happening. I felt as if I were in a war room with generals planning an invasion. The pace was hectic. Typewriters were feverishly clicking away; paralegals and lawyers were filing through massive stacks of documents; documents were being sorted and checked, and were spread over every available surface; people were scrambling everywhere; and groups of lawyers were consulting on different matters. In the middle of this frenzy, the American Osteopathic Association decided to negotiate a settlement rather than go to court, and on October 9, 1980, they agreed to pay us a sum of $30,000 for court costs. They also agreed, in writing, that from that time on they would not do anything to impede professional cooperation between osteopaths and chiropractors.[23] The other defendants, however, held fast.

Our court date was set for December 9. It had taken us seven years to come this far, and now, as tense and even frightening as it was, I wouldn't have had it any other way.

5

THE TEMPEST

Seven years after I first advocated filing a lawsuit against the American Medical Association, and after many struggles with members of my own profession, I sat with Ardith in the empty courtroom, waiting. We both believed that if we succeeded in this battle, it would lead to monumental changes that would better the way health care is delivered in America.

The trial we had prepared for was what was called a simple antitrust lawsuit. "Simple" meant that it was not a class-action lawsuit, but rather a suit on behalf of five individuals. Some of the largest and most prestigious law firms in America represented the defendants. Now we waited for them to come here and paint a proverbial big red bull's-eye on us and attack us in every conceivable way, in hopes of discrediting us as worthwhile doctors, decent citizens, and rational human beings. Our professional files had been carefully scrutinized by a battery of experts who had searched for any improprieties, mistakes, or oversights in our patient histories, x-rays, and other records. We had been subjected to pretrial depositions. Now our adversaries would come after us in court, and we expected them to use every cunning legal trick in the book. All five of us had been warned of this before we got involved, and we had prepared for it ever since; it is the way the game is played. As Harry Truman once said, if you can't stand the heat, you should get out of the kitchen. We had sued them, after all, and they could be expected to do everything possible in self-defense.

The courtroom slowly began to fill. Ardith inclined her head toward me and in a whisper asked if I was nervous. "Yes," I replied, "nervous and excited that this day has finally arrived." I didn't want to put into words how aware I was of everything that was riding on this case—that I had to remain always alert, ever on guard against the tactics of the defense, and as calm as I could be. I wanted to bolster Ardith's spirits with my confidence that this was a fight we could not lose.

A virtual army of lawyers began filing in. Our chief counsel was one of the first to enter, accompanied by a junior partner, Bob Ryan, and Professor Paul Slater. Smiling as he passed me, George stopped momentarily and said, "Well, Chet, this is it!" Those few words said so much to me. We chatted quietly for a few seconds, then he moved toward his position at the right side of the long table.

The stature of this man made him seem to overpower all the others, those who were already in the room and those who continued to file in. He looked right here—the way a star athlete, full of anticipation, looks at the start of a big game. At six feet three inches tall, and weighing about 225 pounds, George McAndrews stood taller and bigger than virtually any other individual in the room; his height, combined with his powerful build and charisma, created an effect that dominated the room. Now in his mid-forties, George was a man who emanated authority and commanded attention. With pride, I felt this was something the defense must see also. The majority of the questioning and cross-examination for our side would be done by George, and his trial experience would be invaluable to us.

A man in his middle thirties took a seat next to George. This was Paul Slater, the professor of antitrust law from Northwestern University who had originally been retained by the NCAC to study the feasibility of bringing this lawsuit. Paul was an academic and he looked like one; he was six feet tall, of medium build, and had brown hair and wore glasses. But Paul was more than just any scholar; he was an expert in antitrust law, and he was considered one of the most brilliant and prominent experts in his field. His understanding of the complexities and intricacies of antitrust law probably surpassed that of all of the other lawyers in the room combined. But he was not a trial attorney *per se*; he was a law professor, and he was here as co-counsel. Just now, the professor appeared nervous and fidgety.

A third individual took a seat near the other two. He was a

man in his late twenties, typically all-American-looking. He appeared almost boyish in this somber room populated mostly by men older than he. He had a round face, hazel-blue eyes, curly brown hair, and a strong physique; he stood about five feet nine and looked clean-cut and athletic, like someone you would see playing handball in a gym. In fact, he said, he had been told by many people that he looked much like the Danno character from the old *Hawaii Five-O* television series. His name was Bob Ryan, and he was not long out of law school—a rookie, comparatively speaking, in George's law firm. He was very likely the youngest lawyer in the room. This case was a training ground for him in antitrust law, a learning experience that few others could equal. Bob was both flattered and a little overwhelmed to be here, in this company. On the one hand, there was George McAndrews, whom he considered to be one of the greatest trial lawyers in America; on the other, there was Paul Slater, whom he regarded as the most outstanding professor of his college career. He had been a student of Slater's at Northwestern, and he said of a group of students there: "We were totally in awe of Paul Slater, and we hung on every word he said. We forgot more of what Paul Slater said than others ever knew."

At hand, within reach of the trio, was a cart laden with file cases. These were stuffed with some of the documents that had been so carefully prepared for use as evidence to support our charges against the American Medical Association and the other fourteen defendants. It would have been impractical to bring into the courtroom all of the 1 million supporting documents that had been gathered, but our legal team had attempted to have ready at hand, filed on this cart, as much of the material as foresight could predict might be needed during the opening phase of the trial. A complete index to all the documents that had been amassed during discovery was also kept as a reference on this cart, so that if any document was needed that had not been brought in, it could be looked up and quickly retrieved.

The courtroom continued to fill. There were so many lawyers representing the various defendants that even though the rectangular table at the front of the courtroom was long, there wasn't room for all of the attorneys to take places across the table from the plaintiffs' legal team. Some of the defense counsel had to sit in chairs along the side of the room. In addition, there were house counsel (lawyers who were regular employees of the defendants) who came to gather information so that they could report the proceedings to their associations' members.

The lawyers representing the defendants were undoubtedly the finest trial lawyers each of the law firms represented had at its disposal. The stakes were high in this case. The American Medical Association was the primary defendant, and it had obviously called out the most experienced of the legal representatives among the law firms it retained for counsel. Our legal representation seemed simple in comparison; it truly looked like a classic David-and-Goliath battle.

The scene inside the courtroom was not much brighter than the gray winter skyscape outside had been. The courtroom was humming, as heads—many of them mature and graying—tilted toward one another in confidential postures. Open briefcases and countless papers were spread all over tables, benches, and carts, and amid the murmuring there was the sound of pages being turned and papers being shuffled. Attorneys and clients were huddled together in a melting pot of legalese, a cauldron beginning to simmer in the heat of the processes of law.

Ardith whispered to me again, "How do you feel about all this?"

I smiled faintly. "I feel good—not just about myself and what's happening, but because I know we're right. We have to prevail. We can't have come to this point after all these years just to fail."

She nodded and stared straight ahead. She didn't want to miss a moment of the action, either.

I took courage from my conviction that George, who had agreed to represent us when no other champion could be found, was in fact the perfect choice for the battle that lay ahead. From the moment he accepted the case, I never doubted, even momentarily, that we would succeed. George was a man who had represented some of the largest corporations in the world. Even more than that, he was totally committed to this cause, regardless of personal consequences. The case he was preparing to prosecute was not one he had undertaken for monetary reasons; in fact, we were the poorest, most ragtag group of clients he ever would agree to represent, and he had no assurance that we would ever raise enough money to pay all our bills. This case was supported as much as possible by voluntary contributions. Beyond that, George himself was our support; he was prepared and willing to write off expenses and fees that could not be paid. And the principal organization he was taking on was a machine with money and political connections that surpassed the scope of anything we could imagine.

We had requested and been granted a trial by jury. Now the jury of eight men and four women entered and took their seats along the side of the room in the section reserved for them. I could feel the excitement and tension building within me.

Finally, Judge Nicholas J. Bua entered the courtroom, and the audience rose to pay him respect. I tried to repress an uneasy feeling I had about this man as the presiding judge. The truth was that I was bothered by our having drawn this particular court-appointed referee, because he had had limited experience with antitrust cases. I had discussed with our attorneys the risks of having a judge with limited experienced in antitrust sitting on the bench and instructing a jury in the intricacies of this special-ized area of the law—even a judge who had a reputation for being extremely bright and a quick learner. Antitrust law is far more complex and difficult to follow than many other fields of law. Lawyers tend to specialize in a specific branch of law (patent and antitrust law, corporate law, criminal law, family law, and so on), and some become brilliant stars who take cases only in their chosen fields, but the same is not true of the judges who hear and decide the cases. The chances of errors being made in the instructions given to the jury are increased when the judge is inexperienced in such cases, and what a jury decides depends heavily on the instructions it receives from the judge. We antici-pated occasional questions of a technical nature, and we hoped that Paul Slater, nationally renowned for his knowledge of anti-trust law, would be allowed to help clarify some of the muddy issues as they arose.

The trial got underway and opening statements were made. Our side, the plaintiffs, went first. George eloquently outlined the case against the defendants and explained the antitrust violations he intended to prove—the intent of the defendants to eliminate chi-ropractic as a competitor; the implementation of that intent with bold action in the form of an elimination program; and the fact that the AMA considered itself successful in its containment and elimination program. His discourse was brilliant! (Later, Judge Bua would comment that George made the finest opening statement he had heard in all the years he had been on the bench.) After George was finished, the defense counsel presented their opening arguments, one after another.

By the time the court recessed for lunch on that first day of the trial, I had decided I did not want to remain in the back of the courtroom any longer. With the complicated legal process involved, I felt like I might miss important points if I sat there. I wanted to hear better and to be closer to the action. Also, it seemed right that I should be closer to my attorney and the rest of the legal team in case they should have any questions that I might be able to answer. So after the noon recess, I moved to one of the front rows, to the left of George, Paul, and Bob. There I stayed for the continuing days of the trial. Ardith continued to sit in the back where, as an observer, she was more comfortable. She said she felt too intimidated by what was happening in the courtroom to move closer, even though I was seated there. Besides that, she said, she felt that she belonged in the back rows. With a smile and a reassuring squeeze of my hand, she promised she would sit in the back and "pray like hell" for George and the others, so that we would all be led to say and do the right things for our cause.

The initial days of the trial were spent introducing a massive number of documents into the court record as evidence, in order to convey to the judge and jury the extent of the antitrust violations. Each document had to be placed in front of the court and introduced into the public record, and the defendants had to be given the opportunity to object to the admission of the evidence if they had a basis for it. This meant that many transcripts of depositions had to be read aloud, so that they would be entered into the court record.

George presented evidence to outline the extent of the AMA's boycott against chiropractic. Notes taken at a meeting of the Michigan State Medical Society (MSMS) meeting in 1973, in which Joseph Sabatier, M.D., of the AMA's Committee on Quackery, compared chiropractors to "rabid dogs" and declared that the AMA considered it "unethical to refer patients to a chiropractor for any purpose whatever," became Plaintiff's Exhibit 1288.[1] (See page 87.) A resolution passed by the MSMS just five days later confirming the MSMS's acceptance of the AMA position became Plaintiff's Exhibit 1291.[2] Another piece of evidence was a letter from the Illinois State Medical Society to the University of Illinois College of Medicine, dated January 11, 1974, which advised:

> It might be wise to prohibit any contact of any kind, at any time, by persons at the Medical Center with any chiropractor.[3]

George then read a letter from the AMA Committee on Quackery to all affiliated medical societies that stated:

> One of the more surprising items brought to the attention of the committee is reported to be professional cooperation and association between Doctors of Medicine and [chiropractors].[4]

The letter went on to instruct the state, local, and specialty societies to inform their members that entering into any professional association with chiropractors was unethical.[5] This letter was also published in the *American Medical News*, a publication sent to all AMA members.[6]

George explained the ostracism of an "unethical" physician in Sedalia, Missouri, Dr. Jerome Block, who was found to be cooperating with a chiropractor, Dr. James Bryden (one of my fellow plaintiffs). He described the way in which Drs. Block and Bryden were compelled to cease to associate professionally—at least openly.[7]

Plaintiff's Exhibit 880 was a letter from a radiologist to a chiropractor containing this statement:

> Since I have not been associated with chiropractic in the past, I felt it necessary to contact the California Medical Association to make sure that our relationship to this time would not be a source of difficulty in the present or future. As it turns out, both the CMA and AMA consider it unethical to associate with chiropractors and, therefore, I will have to reluctantly discontinue performing x-rays on your patients.[8]

And our attorney outlined how the AMA's boycott directly disregarded state legislation on all professional and institutional cooperation. Plaintiff's Exhibit 10A contained a letter dated January 9, 1973, from the Joint Commission on Accreditation of Hospitals to a hospital in New Mexico, which said:

This is in answer to your letter of December 18 referring to a bill which may be passed in New Mexico that hospitals must accept chiropractors as members of the medical staff.

You are absolutely correct—the unfortunate results of this most ill-advised legislation would be that the Joint Commission would withdraw and refuse accreditation of the hospital that had chiropractors on its medical staff.[9]

Further, George presented a letter from the AMA Judicial Council attorney to a member of that organization, in which the AMA evaluated its success with its containment and elimination campaign, saying:

The facts are that chiropractic has not grown in number under existing policy, whereas there is every evidence to believe that it would grow if AMA policy decisions were relaxed.[10]

Document by document, George painted a picture of an intentional, broad-based conspiracy to destroy the chiropractic profession. It took about four weeks to get through all the evidence.

* * *

I started taking notes as I sat in the courtroom on those first days of the trial. I wanted to keep a record for myself of the order of events—what was being said, and by whom. I also thought it would help me to concentrate. When George noticed I was doing this, he said firmly, "Chet, stop taking notes!"

"But," I told him, "if I don't, I won't have them when I need them. I might want to write a book about this someday."

"If necessary, I'll help you with the facts of what happens here," he assured me. "Besides, the court recorder is keeping accurate records of everything. You don't need to."

So, for at least the first week or so, I was able to sit back and listen to all of the testimony, reflect on everything that had happened to bring me here, and consider what I would be able to contribute when my turn came to take the witness stand. That day would come soon enough. Each of the plaintiffs would in fact have his or her day in court. There would come a day for speaking, but now was the time to listen, think, and weigh the arguments, and to try to understand what was happening in the minds of the jury.

I tried to look into the eyes of the jurors and read how they might have been influenced by AMA propaganda, both in the past and now in the courtroom. Probably none of them had any experience with chiropractic (we assumed that if any had, he or she would have been excused from the panel), whereas they all no doubt had consulted medical doctors at one time or another. How unbiased were they really? And could they grasp the complexities of antitrust law? I had read some of the legal briefs in the case myself, and although they were written in English, for all the multisyllabic legalese and complicated points of law, they might as well have been in a foreign language. How could the jury understand them? How could they recognize the relevant facts and separate them from the others? I tried desperately to understand what kind of messages the jury was hearing. And from the early days of the trial, it became clear that certain irrelevant facts were not being kept out of the trial transcripts. Without question, these clouded the antitrust issue.

It was exactly this type of thing we had hoped Paul Slater would be able to head off. For the most part, he sat beside George and passed him notes when he caught something of interest. George did about 95 percent of the talking. Paul's role was more subtle, but he was nevertheless indispensable. He advised George on the fine points, and his expertise in antitrust law was invaluable. He also did do a little bit of the cross-examining of defense witnesses. Occasionally, Paul would stand up and make a point of law. I remember him raising issues to the judge with comments like, "As a point of law, Your Honor, he is wrong. The fact is, in [the name of a case] in [year], this was the decision, and therefore the fact of the law was [such and such]." But brilliant and scholarly as Paul was, the judge often did not take his advice on different points of law.

During a recess early in the trial, I saw Paul Slater in the hallway outside the courtroom. He was impatient with the court's conduct. He was, in fact, furious; his face was red and his body language screamed his frustration. George was trying to calm him down. Paul had been accurately defining the law, but he felt that the court viewed his expert advice as the attempts of a prejudiced advocate to bring out things that favored his own side, rather than as the objective clarifications of a learned professor. He wasn't accustomed to this, and he simply couldn't bear it that the court would not listen to him on points of law. In this place he was no longer the revered professor that he was at Northwestern University, and he was not accorded the same deference. In fact, the court was not at all obliged to accept to his authority on these intricate matters. However, if the court did not understand certain issues, serious errors might be made in the admission of evidence and/or in the jury instructions— which would be sufficient grounds later to call a mistrial.

* * *

George went into the trial without notes. He was such an experienced trial lawyer that he proceeded by instinct. I wondered how he could do this, without even so much as a rough outline. When I asked him, he told me that years before, during his first trial, he had thought he had the whole case worked out in advance. Then the trial got underway. When he asked the first question of his first witness, he got the "wrong" answer—and his entire plan was blown. So he had learned to think on his feet. As our case progressed, he did make his own notes from the court transcripts, and he used those notes along the way.

Interestingly, George had once had a great fear of public speaking. He overcame it by becoming a reader in church. For a couple of years, he read from the Scriptures during services every Sunday to overcome his fright, believing that was the most friendly, compassionate environment he could find in case he stumbled. Then he entered the practice of trial law and had to speak in a courtroom. He told me that during his first case, his knees rattled and his voice warbled like a canary. But the George McAndrews speaking in the courtroom on our behalf was a most confident and articulate attorney.

* * *

Some of the strongest evidence George introduced had to do with the AMA's Committee on Quackery, whose stated goal was no less than the elimination of chiropractic. He produced an outline of the master plan conceived by Robert B. Throckmorton detailing "what medicine should do about the chiropractic menace."[11] Plaintiff's Exhibit 172 was an outline of this plan, which was presented on November 11, 1962, before the North Central Medical Conference in Minneapolis. This master plan provided a strong indictment of the AMA. It drew a complete picture of how the committee leadership had orchestrated the campaign against chiropractic, and how it had proposed to rally national support to make chiropractors look like an incompetent group of people. This document warned that the committee had to conduct its activities "behind the scenes" and "never let [its] hand show" lest it "make the chiropractors underdogs."[12] Portions of the plan advocated and described how to "encourage chiropractic disunity," for example, by having agents attend chiropractic meetings to monitor progress in this regard.[13] Further, it proposed that medical leadership "undertake a positive program of 'containment'" and stated:

> If this program is successfully pursued, it is entirely likely that chiropractic as a profession will "wither and die on the vine" and the chiropractic menace will die a natural but somewhat undramatic death. This policy of containment might well be pursued along the following lines. . . . (4) Encourage ethical complaints against chiropractors. . . . (5) Oppose chiropractic inroads in health insurance. . . . (6) Oppose chiropractic inroads in workmen's compensation. . . . (7) Oppose chiropractic inroads into labor unions. . . . (8) Oppose chiropractic inroads into hospitals. . . . (9) Contain chiropractic schools. . . .
>
> Any action undertaken by the medical profession should be directed toward: . . . (2) Containment of the chiropractic profession. (3) The stifling of chiropractic schools.
>
> Action taken by the medical profession should be . . . (1) Behind the scenes whenever possible. . . .
>
> A successful program of containment will result in the decline of chiropractic.[14]

The intent to contain chiropractic schools, while particularly offensive to us, was basic to the AMA's plan. The document explained this:

> Any successful policy of "containment" of chiropractic, must necessarily be directed at the schools. To the extent that these financial problems continue or multiply, and to the extent that the schools are unsuccessful in their recruiting programs, the chiropractic menace of the future will be reduced and possibly eliminated.[15]

These documents explained why I had been witnessing so many attacks on my profession from so many apparently different sources. They showed clearly how the AMA was orchestrating a well-organized campaign based on a detailed, specific plan for the destruction of chiropractic, and enlisting the help of numerous other medically related organizations and sympathetic individuals. Often, the committee worked covertly, because of concerns that it would be "unwise" to make its activities public.

Some of the other documentation that was admitted for the plaintiffs demonstrated how the AMA had criticized chiropractic's educational base while at the same time taking specific action to harm chiropractic education. For example, Plaintiff's Exhibit 532, an issue of a newsletter published by the Medical Society of the State of New York, provided evidence that when the C.W. Post Center of Long Island University in New York was considering entering into a cooperative program with Lincoln College of Chiropractic, the medical conspirators succeeded in persuading C.W. Post to withdraw its consideration of the proposal.[16] Similar efforts to interfere with the scientific education of chiropractic students were made at Morehead State College in Kentucky and the College of St. Thomas in St. Paul, Minnesota.[17] I found these conspiratorial attacks on the education of an entire group of people to be outrageous, even reminiscent of the infamous book-burning incidents of pre-World War II Europe.

Because the defendants made much of the allegedly inferior education of chiropractors, one day during the trial George suggested something that would have given the jury more understanding about a typical chiropractic education. He proposed to take the entire jury to the National College of Chiropractic in nearby Lombard, Illinois, so that they could see firsthand what a chiropractic education consists of, and honestly assess the quality of the teaching. This college was located less than an hour's drive away, so it would have been simple to charter a bus to take the jury to the college. This would have served to counterbalance the AMA's propaganda, which characterized chiropractic colleges as diploma mills, and to enable the jury to separate fact from fiction; they might observe the classrooms, the laboratories, the x-ray facilities, the anatomy department, the research area, the library, the outpatient clinic, and the administrative offices. They might even visit with instructors. If only the jury could visit the college, I felt, they would see for themselves just how deceitful and dishonest the AMA's propaganda was. Indeed, medical professors have visited this college and remarked that some of its departments were far superior to anything they had ever seen in any medical school.* In my own travels to speak on behalf of chiropractic, I have had the opportunity to see almost every chiropractic college in the United States and England, and I can report with pride that each college seems to be striving to outdo the others in its pursuit of excellence. Chiropractic colleges are accredited by the Council on Chiropractic Education (a federally approved accrediting organization operating under the U.S. Department of Education), in much the same way as medical schools are. In order to be accepted for admission to a four-year chiropractic program at most of these colleges, a student must have a minimum of two years of preprofessional college background. This is a far cry from the image of the uneducated chiropractor promoted by the medical propagandists.

The defense attorneys had been taken on a tour of the National College of Chiropractic before the case went to trial, and they had seen what this college had to offer. When George proposed that the jury visit the college, too, the legal representatives for the defendants proceeded to put up a fight to prevent it, probably because they knew that a properly informed jury would be less likely to decide for their side. Our attorney repeatedly implored the counsel for the defense to change their minds and assent to the visit, but they did not. We then hoped that the judge would order that the jury see the school—in the interest of promoting a greater awareness of the truth—but that did not happen, either. So the jury never had the opportunity to witness what chiropractic education truly is.

On the other hand, the defense was permitted to submit as evidence—over the plaintiffs' strenuous objection—the AMA propaganda book, *At Your Own Risk* by Ralph Lee Smith (see

---

*One such individual was John McMillan Mennell, M.D., a world-renowned doctor and medical school professor who had taught in eight medical schools and visited dozens more as a guest lecturer. At the time of the trial, he was a professor of physical medicine at the University of Connecticut. He visited the National College of Chiropractic and remarked that it had the finest department of anatomy he had ever seen.

page 42). This book was laden with erroneous statements about chiropractic. While it claimed to contain scientific evidence, it was in fact almost totally devoid of any bibliographic references to support its allegations.

On our behalf, Judge Bua did at least admit into evidence the 375-page *Chiropractic in New Zealand Report, 1979*.[18] This report was prepared by the New Zealand Commission of Inquiry as part of an investigation into the desirability of providing benefits for chiropractic care under that government's Social Security and Accident Compensation Acts. It was the result of an inquiry that involved twenty months of study in New Zealand, Australia, Canada, Great Britain, and the United States. The AMA maintained that its actions against the chiropractic profession had been justified because it had been seeking to protect the public against a dangerous cult; the New Zealand report was presented to demonstrate that far from being a dangerous cult, chiropractic was indeed a valuable healing art. Besides exhaustively analyzing the effects (and ultimately the benefits) of chiropractic care, this report thoroughly discredited the propaganda book, *At Your Own Risk*:

> 19. We mention this book [*At Your Own Risk*] simply to show that we have not overlooked it. . . .
> 20. It cannot in the Commission's opinion be regarded as a text on which any reliance can be placed. . . . It is a piece of special pleading. There is no true attempt at objective appraisal of chiropractic. It emphasizes the sensational.
> 21. The author does not appear to have any particular qualifications except the desire to present chiropractic in the worst possible light. The Department of Investigation of the American Medical Association seems to have had something to do with encouraging Smith's investigations; certainly the AMA took a considerable hand in disseminating the book once it was published. It appears to have been published shortly before the United States Senate's Finance Committee's investigation into whether chiropractic treatment should be included in social welfare aid programmes. The Senate Finance Committee disregarded it and so do we.[19]

When it was published in 1979, the New Zealand report was the most comprehensive report that had ever been produced on the subject of chiropractic. The inquiry committee, which consisted of an attorney, a college headmistress, and a professor of chemistry, admitted that in the beginning, it had been prejudiced against chiropractic, but that, "we found ourselves irresistibly and with complete unanimity drawn to the conclusion that modern chiropractic is a soundly based and valuable branch of health care in a specialized area neglected by the medical profession."[20] And in the report's conclusion, the committee stated:

> Modern chiropractic is far from being an unscientific cult. Chiropractors are the only health care practitioners who are necessarily equipped by their training and education to carry out spinal manual therapy.[21]

In his arguments for the plaintiffs, George countered the AMA's claim that its actions were motivated solely by concern for patients with the assertion that economic motives were a factor in the defendants' attacks on chiropractic. A reference to a statement by Dr. Joseph Sabatier at a meeting of the AMA Committee on Quackery was revealing:

> Dr. Sabatier said that the area of alerting the young physicians to the dangers of chiropractic has been neglected—that he [the young M.D.] has the problem of starting a practice, and it would be well to get across the point that the chiropractor is stealing his money.[22]

Another document likewise reflected economic interests. Plaintiff's Exhibit 241 was a letter from an orthopedic surgeon and AMA trustee named Irvin Hendryson that contradicted the organization's public policy and actually admitted to competing with that which they condemned. It concluded:

> Hence, at the University of Colorado we spent a certain amount of time teaching our medical students how to compete with their chiropractic friends across the street.[23]

* * *

An interesting sidelight to the case concerned advice columnist Eppie Lederer (better known by her pen name, Ann Landers). Included in the articles and books she had published were some quite uncomplimentary remarks about chiropractic. Interestingly,

Plaintiff's Exhibit 1407A was a letter from Lederer to Ernest B. (Bert) Howard, M.D., a vice president of the AMA. She wrote:

> Dear Bert:
>
> I know I'll be inundated after my column of August 5th. This man [Robert B. Webb, D.C., a chiropractor who had written a letter to the editor of the *San Francisco Examiner* concerning a column of hers] makes a few good points—(See paragraph 3 and 4).
>
> Can you supply me with a good response, which I will of course rewrite? Many thanks, dear.[24]

The Ann Landers column reached literally millions of faithful readers each and every day. To me, this brought into focus just how pervasive the AMA's antichiropractic propaganda had become.

Another of the allies of the AMA was Professor E.S. Crelin of Yale University. He did not testify in court, but George had spoken with him by telephone prior to the trial. He had published a study, frequently quoted in the medical literature, that purported to be a test of chiropractic theory.[25] In this study, he looked in fresh cadavers for evidence of the type of vertebral subluxations or vertebral dysfunction to which chiropractors refer, and did not find any. This much-cited study, however, was completely worthless, for two very important reasons. First of all, Crelin had decided ahead of time what the outcome would be. In a letter dated January 24, 1972—that is, *before* his study even began—he wrote:

> I have purchased the necessary equipment and I am now setting up experiments to blow their profession [chiropractic].[26]

Second, the entire project was based on a faulty concept: A subluxation can no more occur in a cadaver than you can slap a ham and cause swelling. A subluxation complex is both a physiological and structural dysfunction, and can occur only in a living body.

* * *

Shortly before the trial began, the American Osteopathic Association had decided to settle out of court with us. The Chicago Medical Society—whose leaders and attorneys had insisted that there were medical officers within the CMS who had been deal-ing with chiropractors all along—now also decided to settle.[27] That left thirteen defendants to face as the trial wore on.

6

THE EYE OF THE STORM

As the weeks went by, I sat in the courtroom and watched as various individuals were called to take the witness stand. The time would soon come for me to do the same. I recalled my days as a high school student, and remembered well the gripping fear I had experienced once when I had had to stand up before my English class to give a speech. I had known for a month beforehand which day I would be scheduled to speak, and with growing dread I counted the days. As the fateful day approached, I fantasized about cutting class, but brushed the idea aside, knowing that it would only have postponed the inevitable. Besides, it would have drawn more attention to my speech—I would have had to make up the missing assignment on another day, when no one else would be speaking. The environment in class had been a friendly one, but even so, the prospect of speaking publicly was crippling to me.

By the time I was in college, I felt a little better about speaking in public. But even then, it took effort on my part simply to raise my hand to ask questions of the instructors. I avoided asking questions whenever possible. Often, I would sit and wait until the last possible moment, hoping that somebody else would ask the question that I was thinking of, so I wouldn't have to.

Since then, of course, I had found it necessary to develop my abilities as a public speaker. In the course of writing *Chiropractic Speaks Out*, I had become completely convinced that the only solution to the dilemma facing chiropractic was effective mass communication. Our profession needed articulate chiropractors who were equipped and able to counteract the propaganda put out by the AMA's war machine. Chiropractic needed to communicate accurate, up-to-date information, and someone would have to take the lead in showing us how. I was quite outside of my own comfort zone in doing this; at first, invitations to speak at chiropractic conventions or on radio and TV talk shows and interviews profoundly intimidated me. But when the going gets tough, the tough must get going. I vowed that if it took the rest of my life, I would do what I could to help bring truth and honesty to health care. Even if standing at a speaker's podium made my knees quake, I was sure enough of my information to deliver the message. Besides, by this time my fear of speaking had largely been replaced with anger at what I witnessed from the AMA and its allies—combined with disgust at the leaders of my own profession, who were doing so little to correct the lies. With a little practice, I adapted surprisingly quickly to what had once been the paralyzing nightmare of public speaking, and I even learned to enjoy it and consider it a privilege.

Now here I was, preparing to take the witness stand in the presence of a judge, facing a courtroom full of lawyers. The chief counsel of major law firms would be bent on destroying my credibility as a witness, and probably as a doctor and a rational human being as well. Every word I uttered would be duly and diligently recorded by the court stenographer, and the transcripts would subsequently be studied by fiercely critical experts whose job was to find ways to attack and undermine my testimony. If anyone had ever suggested to me that the day would come when I would actually look forward to this experience with relish, I would have considered them crazy, sure that there was no way I ever would or could—yet, strangely, I now found that I did.

What made the difference was my cause. The faces of the medical representatives in this place were not like that of the friendly family physician most of us know from our own personal experience. These men were a different breed altogether; they were people who wielded control of the largest and most powerful medical organization in the world, and who influenced satellite organizations as well, and they had injured a great many people by their blind ambition. My outrage at their power and greed gave me a motivating energy unlike anything I had known before. It gave me the strength to do what had to be done.

I considered the various depositions that I had been required to give, and I wondered which material might be used in an attempt to discredit me and the case. George himself had prepared me to testify. Arguably the finest antitrust trial lawyer in America, George knew what kinds of ploys the AMA and other defendants' attorneys might use in their arguments. I remained firm in my conviction that we were right and that, in the American system of justice, truth would prevail.

As it happened, I did not spend as much time on the witness stand as I had expected. For the most part, I was asked innocuous questions, similar to those I had been asked before. However, two subjects were brought up that stand out in my mind in such a way that I am sure I will never forget them.

The first concerned a patient I had treated over a one-year period. Max Wildman, the lead attorney for the AMA, focused on the fact that I had seen this patient approximately 100 times during the year I treated him. The implication was that I had exploited this poor patient by recommending excessive treatment. The attorney framed his comments in such a way that I could not respond defensively to them. He knew well that if I were given the opportunity to explain the situation, I could void his attempt to make me look like a greedy fraud.

The patient in question was a sweet senior citizen in his eighties. Tony stood under five feet tall, because he had absolutely the most severe scoliosis (a spinal curvature) that I had ever seen. If not for the scoliosis, he would have been much taller, perhaps five feet five inches. By trade, Tony was a building inspector, and we used to joke that if his spine were a building, it would have been condemned and torn down long ago. His wife was an invalid, and the cost of her care kept him broke financially and dependent on being able to continue to work. He had Medicare coverage, and I agreed to treat him and accept whatever Medicare would pay. There was a limit on the number of treatments that Medicare would cover, and Tony's own private insurance gave poor coverage, so the end result was that I treated him for almost nothing—I probably averaged less than two dollars per treatment from him over the year. I just wrote off whatever the insurance plans did not pay.

Tony told me he believed the chiropractic adjustments were the only thing in this world that kept him going—that without them he would have been dead and buried many years before. He insisted on coming in for adjustments twice a week. During blizzards in Chicago, when all my other patients would cancel their appointments, Tony never did—rain, snow, or shine, he would always make it in to see me. How could anyone turn such a person away? I believe the lawyer questioning me knew the circumstances of the case. Indeed, he had asked my receptionist, Edna Kehm, why I had treated Tony for practically no charge, and she had responded, "Because Dr. Wilk has a good heart." But even so, the AMA attorney presented the case in such a way that a humane act was twisted to look like a sign of greed. No doubt his intention was to rock me off balance, and he did exactly that.

Out of the corner of my eye, I saw the jury, and I knew I had no way to let them know the truth about this case; the line of questioning left them with conclusions that I had no opportunity to refute. I later asked George to put me back on the stand and direct the questioning so as to set the record straight, but he didn't feel it would be worth doing that for the purpose of making a single point, and I trusted his judgment.

The other line of cross-examination I remember well was used by another of the AMA attorneys, Doug Carlson. He asked me about the communication seminars I conducted for chiropractors around the country.

"Now, Dr. Wilk," he asked, "by the way, do you teach courses to chiropractors on how to answer questions?"

I answered, "I teach courses on how chiropractors can answer questions accurately and effectively, keeping [their answers] in the proper context."

"And have you been using some of the teachings in your courses as you answered my questions today?"

"If you mean trying to give honest, accurate answers—yes, I have."

Carlson then rephrased the question. "Have you been using the teachings in your courses today, sir? That is my question."[1]

I had created an audiotape series to teach chiropractors to be better communicators of the chiropractic message, and to enable them to present this message to the media, in courtroom testimonies, and in patient communication. I had also conducted roundtable communication meetings with doctors of chiropractic. I did all this because of certain serious failures I had observed in chiropractic communication. Most of these problems stemmed from the fact that chiropractors, although they meant well, often used techniques that did not accurately or appropriately communicate their message. For example, some terms that were in common use among those in the profession (things that might be called chiropractic jargon) tended to sound strange and unfamiliar to the general public. Instead of truly communicating just what it is that chiropractors do, they simply created more problems. The medical propagandists used some of these phrases, which tended to sound more spiritual than scientific, to embarrass chiropractic. I believed that if chiropractic could deliver its message accurately and understandably, it would achieve widespread public acceptance. In my view, public misunderstanding—most of it the result of medical propaganda—had been by far the greatest stumbling block to chiropractic. Public ignorance was the root of the problem, and chiropractors needed to learn effective methods of communicating the truth about what we do. Then there would be no holding chiropractic back!

The lawyers cross-examining me were well aware of my stand on this issue, because I had explained it to them in the process of giving my previous depositions. They knew that all I was trying to do was to teach chiropractors to avoid playing into the hands of adversarial attorneys or people in the media. Yet had I simply answered, "Yes" at this point, I anticipated the AMA attorney would have said something like, "Thank you, Dr. Wilk. No further questions." Of course, the inference would have been that I was a slick operator and that the jury should not be taken in by any of my answers. I saw this coming a mile away. To avoid setting myself up to be a victim of this trick, I decided to qualify my answer.

And so I explained that I was indeed using techniques from my course insofar as they helped me to really listen to the questions and answer them in their proper context—so that I wouldn't be led into saying something contrary to what I was actually thinking. "Because I'm sure you know," I said, "that an adversary attorney will oftentimes ask leading questions which will distort the real meaning of what the person is trying to answer."

Not at all happy with my answer, the attorney popped back quickly by asking me, in effect, if I was accusing him of doing this. "Now, Dr. Wilk," he admonished, "do you have any doubt that your attorney and the judge here will not allow me to distort anything?"

Of course, the answer to that too was yes, but again I hesitated for a moment as I thought of exactly which words I should use to answer. The AMA attorney, meanwhile, must have realized immediately that this was not a question that would serve his cause, because before I could say anything in reply, he quickly said, "I will withdraw the question." At this, Judge Bua looked up at him and asked, "Aren't you afraid to get an answer to that?" and the courtroom erupted in laughter.[2]

* * *

The other plaintiffs were questioned as well. Their testimony primarily concerned the ways in which they personally had been affected by the AMA boycott. James Bryden, the plaintiff from Sedalia, Missouri, was a balding man with a thin, almost skeletal-looking face. Despite his unimposing appearance, he refused to be intimidated and endured well under the scrutiny of the attorneys. In fact, he had looked forward to going to court and making public the injustices perpetrated against him and his patients by the medical establishment. He was outraged because the local hospital had attempted to prevent him from referring patients with suspected heart trouble to a cardiologist—in effect, preventing him from providing his patients with appropriate health care—and this made him a strong voice on behalf of the case challenging the AMA's boycott of chiropractic.

Dr. Mike Pedigo, a big, burly man, had been extremely concerned about saying something improper or inaccurate while on the witness stand. But if he was at all uneasy, he did not look it. He had asked a local hospital for the privilege of referring patients for radiology services in cases he felt needed additional x-ray evaluation. The hospital turned him down, and when he learned that the primary reason was the AMA boycott, he was furious. In effect, he said, his patients had been denied appropriate health care services because he was a doctor of chiropractic.

Pat Arthur, the chiropractor-plaintiff whose experience with the boycott had ultimately cost her her practice in Colorado (see page 78), was a tall, distinguished-looking woman with silvery blonde hair. In the courtroom she maintained her composure both under George's direct examination, as she recounted the story of what had been done to her, and under extremely tough cross-examination by the defendants' attorneys. Despite the great emotion and stress she must have felt, she never let it show in court, even when the defense attorneys seemed to be trying their hardest to get to her. She was a most courageous plaintiff.

* * *

Among the most interesting items entered into evidence by the defense were from a file that the AMA had accumulated containing a copy of every letter that I had ever mailed to any chiropractic association. Actually, I found their decision to submit items from this file as evidence puzzling, because if anything, it seemed to me that its very existence tended to support allegations of conspiracy. The fact was, the AMA had a better record of every piece of correspondence that I had ever sent than I had! Some of the letters I did not even have copies of; sometimes, when I had run short of photocopied letters, I would mail out my last one. There must have been people on the inside of the national and state chiropractic associations who were also in league with the AMA, and who diligently kept them informed of my progress in trying to enlist help for the lawsuit—just as the quackery committee's internal memos had instructed them to do.[3] Had I even suspected that this might be the case, I would have coded my letters in some way so that the source of the espionage could have been traced. But this dossier proved how well organized was the AMA's monitoring of every little bit of progress for the cause of chiropractic.

The question then begged to be asked: If the AMA was, on the one hand, so well informed about every letter I wrote to enlist support for the antitrust suit, how could it, on the other hand, be so grossly ignorant of the many studies proving the effectiveness and superiority of chiropractic treatment for certain health problems? In my opinion, this was a paradox. When it came to gathering information about chiropractic, the AMA was, on the one hand, most cunning and well informed, and on the other, conveniently ignorant.

* * *

One of the defense's primary arguments was that chiropractic was an unscientific cult that relied more on business techniques, which often bordered on fraud, than on any useful therapeutic methods. To justify this position, the defendants dwelled very heavily on a so-called practice management course taught by Dr. James Parker, a chiropractor in Dallas, Texas. They submitted as evidence one of his earliest publications—long since out of date—and offered it as evidence of unethical teachings advanced by chiropractors. Specifically, it contained advice on how to attract patients and emphasized the potential profitability of a chiropractic practice. Despite the fact that this material was thoroughly obsolete and reflected little or nothing of modern chiropractic, not a single day of the trial passed without that practice management book being on the bench where the plaintiffs' attorneys sat, so that it was in plain view of the jury. The defense attorneys often picked it up and used it to argue that chiropractic was more of a money-oriented business than a health-oriented profession, and to help justify the AMA's attempt to destroy chiropractic.

This is not to say that I would have defended the content of the material. Some of the practices it spoke of were not in the best of taste, and the profit motive was indeed overemphasized. But besides being entirely outdated, this material had absolutely no place in the evidence of a simple antitrust lawsuit, and it was used for one purpose only: to influence the minds of the jury against the chiropractor-plaintiffs. In courtroom battle, anything may be tried as long as the court permits it.

I found it particularly maddening, and endlessly frustrating, that the defendants continued to reiterate the argument that chiropractic is unscientific and to force this as an issue. In fact, every M.D. who took the witness stand was given the opportunity to give some example demonstrating that chiropractic does *not* work, and none could. George had told them in advance that this question would be coming, and they had ample time to consult with their medical colleagues and search for such a case. Each time George asked the question, he held his breath, knowing that the doctors had had every opportunity to prepare an answer. Yet no one was ever able to give the proof he asked for. This illustrated the double standard that existed—and that still exists—for medicine and chiropractic. Proof that chiropractic does not work in cases of vertebral or structural dysfunction apparently does not exist. Proof that medicine does not work in such cases *does* exist, but it is generally ignored, and most people never give it a second thought.

Yet the words "scientific" and "unscientific" were constantly repeated, in all of the briefs and pleadings of the AMA and the other defendants. Besides the fact that the underlying assumption—that chiropractic was unscientific—was untrue and could be disproved, the scientific basis of the profession was in fact irrelevant because it was not at issue in the case. The issue was the antitrust actions of the AMA and the other defendants. But the defendants continued to declare chiropractic invalid and to use this assertion as a justification for their own improper conduct. Their attorneys kept harping on the material in the practice management book that focused on making money, said that it proved chiropractic to be quackery, and professed that the defendants had been seeking only to eliminate quackery. They also brought up cases of questionable conduct on the part of certain individual chiropractors. Yet just as the scientific basis of chiropractic was really irrelevant to the case, so too the ethics of individual chiropractors was not at issue. Paul Slater attempted to make it clear to the court that neither science nor ethics had relevance in an antitrust case—that antitrust is a legislative matter protecting trade and commerce from unlawful restraints, monopolies, and unfair business practices—but the court was not listening, and I could see signs that the constant references to the practice management material were prejudicing the jury against chiropractic.

* * *

We were now approaching a part of the trial that I was particularly eager to see—when the defendants' lawyers would bring in H. Doyl Taylor, director of the AMA's Department of Investigation and the secretary of the AMA Committee on Quackery. He was the man who had been responsible for so much of the written propaganda, and who orchestrated the maneuverings of the elimination committee. I wanted to see him face to face, look him straight in the eye, and see if he could look back at me. I hoped to define just what had so possessed this man that he would dedicate twelve years of his life to trashing our profession. What kind of person would devote his life to such dishonesty? I wondered if he would squirm and perspire under scrutiny, like his old friend and associate on the quackery committee, Dr. Sabatier, had done when I debated him once on a radio talk show in New Orleans.

On a Friday afternoon, I learned that Doyl Taylor was scheduled to appear the following Monday morning. All weekend I anticipated what the next day of the trial would bring. I had no idea if I would say anything to Taylor when I saw him. But I considered it well worth the wait and the many years of hassle to finally come to this event.

I eagerly made the trip downtown on the day Taylor was scheduled to testify in court. Again that day, I was the first one to arrive in the courtroom. I did not want to miss one minute of this day. I waited as George and the usual pack of defense lawyers filed into the courtroom. And I kept looking around, expecting at any moment to see the nefarious Doyl Taylor make his appearance. The minutes ticked past, but he did not appear.

The proceedings began, and still he had not arrived. The defendants appeared calm, not the least bit apprehensive. And then it was announced that Taylor was not going to appear. Without notice, he had moved out of Chicago the Friday before the trial started! He had taken his ailing wife and moved to Arizona. He had left the jurisdiction of the Northern Illinois Federal Court, leaving us without the witness I had most looked forward to seeing here.

I thought, My God! He's running like a scared rat! He was so quick to trash our profession with his propaganda, but now he won't step forward to face the judge and jury. If he was so eager to attack us, why not meet us face to face in court? I had come, as had the other three plaintiffs, prepared to answer whatever the defendants' attorneys had to throw at us, but where was Doyl Taylor, the man who had so totally committed himself to our demise?

Doyl Taylor's son did come to the courtroom. Under oath, he testified that his father had crippling arthritis and was physically unable to come to Chicago to testify.

In response, our defense team hired a detective agency in Arizona to investigate, and to see if Taylor really was as ill as his son had testified. We learned that he was regularly spending time on the golf course. Clearly, playing golf would not be a normal pastime for a man who had crippling arthritis. Included in the report we received from the detective agency was an account that once, while going into a convenience store for a cup of coffee, the private investigator working on our case accidentally bumped into Taylor, who was coming out. The two of them exchanged polite words of apology, and according to the investigator, Taylor seemed fine. I found it disappointing and a breach of the public interest that the jury was prevented even from knowing that despite the arthritis that made him "too ill" to travel back to Chicago to testify, Doyl Taylor was actually healthy enough to play golf nearly every day.

* * *

During a court recess one day, our legal team, the other plaintiffs, and I were having a conversation about the way things were going, when Paul Slater said something that was, at that moment, the finest, most heartwarming tribute we could have been given. Coming from a professional of Paul's caliber, it was especially meaningful, and perhaps that is why I remember it. He said that when representing major corporations in antitrust litigation, he had seen ruthless, self-interested corporations going after each other with such a vengeance that it was hard to get emotionally involved with any of them. But in this case, he told me, he felt like he was on the side of the angels.

* * *

I was in the courtroom almost every day of the trial. I had retained another chiropractor to see my patients in the office during the daytime when I would be in court. The court sessions convened at ten o'clock in the morning, recessed for lunch, then resumed at one in the afternoon. In midafternoon, around two or three o'clock, I would leave for my office, which was about a forty-five-minute commute from downtown. Of course, I saw fewer patients during those weeks, given my abbreviated office schedule, but the clinic did not have to cut back on the overall number of patients. I know that the change in the attending doctor did cause some patients to drift away. Some people do not like change, and prefer to see only a doctor to whom they are accustomed. In addition, I had many patients who were immigrants from Poland, and my not being available to answer the telephone when a Polish-speaking person called caused me to lose a few patients. Also, a large portion of my energy was going into the trial instead of the practice. While the impact on my practice was not favorable, it was worth it to me. I had fought for years to get the suit started, and when it finally was under-way, it was an answer to my prayers.

But now the trial was drawing to a close, and I had an uneasy feeling about the turn it had taken. Some of the evidence that had been admitted for the defense was irrelevant and should never have been admitted into the court record in a simple antitrust lawsuit—especially the "practice management" material (see page 134), portions of which had been taken out of context so that it was made to look worse than it was. By association, we chiropractor-plaintiffs were being made to appear more interested in making money than in the welfare of our patients.

While this material was entered into evidence, other items were not. Particularly damaging, I felt, was the fact that my book, *Chiropractic Speaks Out: A Reply to Medical Propaganda, Bigotry and Ignorance* (see page 41), was never admitted as evi-dence. This book had been written specifically to expose (and correct) the misinformation being spread about chiropractic, and it had been mentioned in a deposition read by one of the defense attorneys during the trial. This should have made it possible to introduce it to the jury as evidence, and George made numerous attempts to do so. But one or another of the lawyers for the defense would always object to it, and the judge never permitted its admission.

It seemed clear to me that the real issue in the case was being obscured. Matters specifically relevant to the antitrust issue (rather than the relative merits of medicine and chiropractic) were not allowed to be heard and therefore could not be considered by the jury. In this simple antitrust lawsuit, the essential question was whether or not the defendants had illegally conspired to contain and eliminate chiropractic—not the specifics and/or success rate of chiropractic treatment. I often felt impossibly frustrated as I witnessed the various attorneys' theatrics. There seemed to be a lot more fanfare than substance in the material the defense attorneys presented. In my mind, the jury was being manipulated, and were by design the most ignorant and misinformed people in that courtroom. In the closing days, as I looked into the eyes of the jury, I had the feeling that they were simply not aware of what really mattered here. I hoped I was wrong.

One morning, as I prepared to leave for the courtroom, Ardith asked the unthinkable: "What if the jury doesn't see it our way, and we lose the case?"

I replied, "That just can't happen. We can't fail, because we won't quit until we win this and expose the lies and the fraud for what they are. It's only a matter of how long it will take." I was convinced, but how could I convince her? I had learned one thing early in life, and had been repeatedly reminded of it: No man is an island. Eventually, we must all must answer for the ways in which we have hurt others. Someday, somehow, right would prevail. And I was committed to stay with it until that happened.

* * *

The trial lasted seven weeks. For eight weeks, Bob Ryan barely got any sleep—he averaged only about four hours a night. He spent hours on the case, working well into the night, both in his office and at his home. Fifteen lawyers were trying to keep our team of three attorneys busy and throw them off balance with the filing of motions and requests to change the schedule of witnesses. In fact, during the second half of the trial, when the defense presented its case, it seemed that the lawyers for the defense were constantly changing the order in which their witnesses would appear in court. Our attorneys would prepare to cross-examine an announced witness on the day before he or she was to appear, and then the defendants would change who would be appearing at the last moment. This forced our lawyers to stay up half the night preparing for a different witness. During the presentation of the defendants' case, this happened almost daily—sometimes two or three times in one day. This created great problems for our attorneys, particularly Bob. And behind the scenes, Bob was also writing necessary motions and briefs.

Eventually, the trial came to a close. When the court adjourned, at five o'clock in the afternoon on January 30, 1981, we all went home to wait for the jury's verdict.

The next day, I called George's office. The switchboard operator told me that George was not in the office, and she offered to take a message for him. Then she told me that the jury had returned a verdict in our case. They had deliberated for only two hours, and the defendants had been found *not guilty.* My worst fear had been realized.

7

QUIET AFTER THE STORM

While our defeat was a loss for us, I believed it meant a graver loss to the thousands of people who die every year from complications due to unnecessary surgeries and reactions to medications. This fight had been undertaken on behalf of those people as well as on behalf of chiropractic. It was indeed a fight for the millions of patients who were being victimized by the boycott against chiropractic.

* * *

In January of 1976, the medical doctors in Los Angeles County went on strike. State audits later concluded that during that month, the death rate there *dropped*, possibly by as many as 153 people, as a result of the amount of elective surgery that was not performed.[1]

Leighton Cluff, M.D., a U.S. Public Health Service epidemiologist, conducted a study at Johns Hopkins University in 1964. He found that of all the people who were hospitalized at Johns Hopkins' Osler Service over a three-month period, approximately 14 percent had their stays prolonged because of medication reactions.[2] Dr. William Boyd, one of America's most renowned pathologists, and author of *A Textbook of Pathology: An Introduction to Medicine*, criticized the excessive use of medications.[3] He said that allergies to drugs were increasing to epidemic levels that would soon exceed bacterial disease in number.[4] His implied advice was that if we continued to fool with nature, we would have to pay the penalty. As far as medications were concerned, he wrote, "What is powerful for good can be potent for evil."[5]

Elihu M. Schimmell, M.D., conducted a survey at the Yale New Haven Hospital over an eight-month period in 1963. Dr. Schimmell was chief resident at the hospital, which is connected with the Yale University School of Medicine. He was interested in iatrogenic— doctor-caused—illnesses, and his question was how often medical treatment, both diagnostic and therapeutic, actually creates or worsens illness, or results in death. Dr. Schimmell studied information reported by thirty-three staff doctors concerning 1,014 hospital patients, and he determined that as many as 20 percent of them suffered complications as a result of the medical care they received in the hospital.[6] "One in five of the patients was made ill by medical treatment, and it caused or contributed significantly to more than one in ten of all hospital deaths," he reported.[7] Extrapolating from his conclusions, one might estimate, conservatively, that there were more than 5 million doctor-caused diseases annually, and that 100,000 American people died in hospitals each year from "noxious episodes" (reactions to medications) alone—a rough average of 2,000 deaths a week.[8]

There is ample evidence that the situation has not improved since Dr. Schimmell did his famous study. In 1985, Dan Rather reported on a study showing that some 180,000 people die every year as a result of hospital errors.[9] In 1990, Dean Howard Hiatt of Harvard University published a study concluding that in one year alone, medical negligence had resulted in 99,000 injuries and 7,000 deaths among hospital patients—and that was just in New York state.[10] In July of 1993, consumer advocate Ralph Nader released an even more alarming study pointing to "a virtual epidemic of medical malpractice" in America.[11] According to this study, between 150,000 and 300,000 Americans are injured or killed each year as a result of medical negligence that occurs in hospitals. This is the numerical equivalent of one fully loaded jumbo jet for each day of the year, and it does not include people who suffer doctor-caused injury outside of the hospital setting. Further, some 80,000 people die each year as a result of medical negligence. That is twice the annual number of traffic fatalities in this country, and roughly 22,000 more than died in the entire course of the Vietnam War.[12] And every one of the individuals who died left anguished, bereaved loved ones. It is mind-boggling to think that all of these deaths were *unnecessary*, and they occurred in the name of "modern" medicine.

All of these numbers, I believe, hold a solemn message for us.

Unfortunately, however, we too often are prone to overlook even the clearest of messages. Winston Churchill summarized this when he said, "Man trips over the truth and then just keeps on walking as though nothing had happened." How tragically correct he was!

Our courtroom battle had been a fight to bring light into the darkness of the American health care system and to achieve closer interprofessional cooperation among health care disciplines. This could only help to reduce the staggering number of deaths. We had lost our case, but that loss was small compared with these statistics and with the pain of the grieving families. These people were the victims of a situation that had to be changed if we were ever to have rational, safe, effective, and unrestricted health care in this country.

Our loss was a loss for free choice, too. We were confronting a national health care crisis of major proportions that needed to be properly addressed. Simply put, this crisis was one of ignorance and prejudice in health care, and it was costing the lives of thousands of victims of unnecessary surgery and iatrogenic reactions. Antitrust violations hurt every one of us in ways we don't really even think about or understand.

* * *

Many of us have someone we look up to as a hero and mentor. For years, I had regarded Winston Churchill as my inspiration. I had been fascinated by this most unusual man, who lived at a critical time in history and made a profound difference. He was a model of strength and persistence to me—a real bulldog, as he was often called.

Churchill was not an obvious choice to become one of the greatest communicators, military leaders, and statesmen the world has ever known. He was short, fat, and bald, and he had a speech impediment—a stutter. Winston Churchill didn't have the looks or the bearing of a leader. But people recognized him as a genius. This man was able to rally England and the Allied forces against a foe darker than any the world had ever seen, at a time when the future looked most bleak. His genius was in his ability to communicate and to press onward—to persevere and refuse to be beaten. He did not know defeat; it was a word that did not exist for him.

That portrait of persistence encouraged me to find strength to carry on in the darkest moments of the struggle. And the period after we lost the trial was the bleakest time I had known.

What would Churchill have said in a situation like this? I wondered. And then I reflected upon a time when Churchill, then an elder statesman, was called upon once again to speak to Parliament on the pressing issues of the day. The members of Parliament had come prepared to stay through the night, if necessary, to hear the wisdom Churchill would have for them. Parliament was packed, but as he approached the podium, such a hush fell over the assembly that you could have heard a pin drop. Then Winston Churchill spoke.

"Never give up!" he said. And then, increasing his volume, and with all the fire and tenacity for which he was known, he added, "Never, ever give up!" And with this, he turned away and sat down in his seat. Those seven words were all he uttered. He startled and mesmerized the entire Parliament with those brief words.

If Churchill had been here to offer us advice, I believed, those would have been his words to us, too. I had to believe that in our democracy, those who have persistence and who champion the truth are ultimately destined to prevail.

* * *

The switchboard operator who had informed me of the verdict in our case had also told me that George lost his voice temporarily the day after the verdict was reached. Mike Pedigo was with George when the verdict was announced. He told me that George took it very hard that night and that his disappointment was profound. By the following morning, however, after a good night's sleep, George's disappointment had turned into anger, and he set to work preparing to file an appeal.

I finally got to speak at length with George when he came over to my home for an adjustment. Afterwards, we stayed up rather late, talking in my kitchen, and he was his usual positive and committed self. He seemed undaunted by the defeat and ready to carry on with the same intensity. Of course, I never doubted him for one second. I knew how committed he was to this cause, and if he had ever had a thought of quitting, I never knew it and he was well beyond it now.

He said to me, "Chet, doesn't it seem that nothing of great importance in life ever seems just to fall into place? These are the things that must be pioneered. Only those who never give up ultimately accomplish their goals. We are the pioneers who must persist in this." It was an uplifting conversation, and we agreed on what needed to be done.

And then George told me of an interesting development. After the trial was over, he had received an unexpected telephone call from one of the jurors, who was in tears. She told him that she had not been able to sleep all night after the verdict was in; she said she had cried all night. George told her that he would not be able to speak to her, since this call was most inappropriate, but she went on, saying, "What the AMA did was very wrong, but you know, Mr. McAndrews, some of those chiropractors should have gone to jail!"

The juror was referring not to the chiropractor-plaintiffs, but to the people mentioned in the practice-building material that the AMA had dwelled upon so heavily during the trial. In other words, the jury had based its decision not on antitrust issues at all, but on irrelevant material they should never have seen in the first place! It created a backlash of jury sympathy, and a desire among the jurors to right, in a public way, isolated wrongs of bad taste and questionable or unethical practices. Apparently, this was a major factor that led to our losing the lawsuit.

* * *

While the chiropractic profession was extremely disappointed, and some members of it even shocked, by the jury's verdict, the defeat was not as bad as it might have seemed. All the documents we had gathered during the discovery phase had been worthless to us until they became part of the public record. Among these were the documents that had originally surfaced from Sore Throat, as well as those that been printed in the underground publication *In the Public Interest*. Until they had been established as genuine, they were of no legal value to our case. During the discovery phase, George had searched through great numbers of documents in the files at AMA headquarters, to extract the evidence we needed to build our case. We had, in fact, been successful in entering substantial numbers of documents important to the support of our case into the public record of the federal court. The proof of our claims was indelibly recorded. This had been a principal objective, and in successfully achieving it, we had achieved victory in at least one of our important goals.

True, the case had been lost. But if we mounted a successful appeal, the suit would be remanded back to the district court to be heard by a new judge. We had lost the battle, but the war was not over.

Once we decided to appeal, the next step was to take the decision to the United States Court of Appeals for the Seventh Circuit to file the case for appeal. Then we waited. These matters take a great deal of time, and ultimately a lot of time is spent waiting.

George prepared most of the paperwork for the appeal by himself, without any help from his legal support staff, and he filed the appeal himself, too. Because we had lost the first case and because there was a severe shortage of money, he could not use the resources of his law firm to get this work done. Secretaries and clerks have to be paid, after all. So he did as much as was feasible by himself. This was our lowest ebb, both financially and psychologically.

On November 21, 1981, the American Academy of Physical Medicine and Rehabilitation settled with us out of court. This is not a large organization, and no doubt they were interested in drawing a line on the fees being charged for legal services. The appeals process is a very time-consuming and costly one. Also, no doubt, they saw the intensity of our commitment to win this battle.

That left the AMA and eleven other defendants named in our plea for an appeal.

Finally, three years after George filed the appeal, the time came for our attorneys to bring our request for a new trial before a panel of three judges. In order for the lawsuit to stay alive, we had to win.

It was January of 1982. The courtroom was packed to overflowing, standing room only, and people who were unable to get in were standing in the hall outside. There was barely breathing room. I was lucky to get inside the courtroom that day, and I wouldn't have but for the fact that I was a plaintiff in the case. The AMA and its allies, the eleven other defendants who remained, knew—as we did—that this was a critical phase of the suit. If they won here, reversing the previous ruling would be extremely difficult, if not impossible. As a last resort, a final appeal before the Supreme Court of the United States might be made available to us, but the odds there were heavily against even being heard. On the other hand, if the AMA and its allies lost here, it would breathe new life into our case, and we would get a second chance with the lower district court. The stakes were high.

George presented our case before the three-judge panel, arguing that the court had made multiple mistakes in issuing directions during the trial and in instructing the jury at the trial's end. In its study of the transcripts of the first trial, our legal team had counted thirteen errors on the part of the district court, giving us room for what lawyers call "throwaways." In other words, there were so many points on which the case could be reversed that even if some of them were thrown out, we could still win. Our hopes were high that the case would be sent back to the district court.

One of the judges asked George, "Are you saying that the trial was conducted under massive error?"

Without hesitation, George replied, "Yes, Your Honor." In my seat, I nodded my head in silent agreement. As far as I was concerned, that was an understatement, to say the least.

The hearing came to an end, and once again, all we could do was go home to wait for the verdict. And once again, we clung to our hopes that the decision would be a favorable one.

It seemed as if we were waiting forever, but this time I felt more confident. Finally, on September 19, 1983, the U.S. Court of Appeals for the Seventh Circuit handed down their verdict: The three-judge panel unanimously agreed that there had indeed been massive error on the part of the lower court in instructing the jury in the case of *Wilk v. AMA*, and it reversed the judgment of that court (which had been based upon the jury's verdict) and ordered a new trial for the chiropractor-plaintiffs. In a forty-seven-page judgment, the case was sent back for retrial, with very specific directions on the law to be applied.[13] On December 1, 1983, the Court of Appeals denied all of the defendants' requests that it reconsider its ruling. We were given one more chance to retry the case at the lower district level.

* * *

Having made a careful analysis of the legal issues, the appeals court set the ground rules for a "patient care defense," which the AMA and other defendants would have to satisfy at retrial. That is, even if the plaintiffs established that an otherwise illegal combination in restraint of trade (an illegal monopoly) did exist, the AMA and other defendants would nevertheless be excused and held not liable under the Sherman Act if they could show:

1. That their opposition to chiropractic was genuinely motivated by a concern for the use of proper scientific method in the treatment of patients.
2. That this concern was objectively reasonable.
3. That this concern was the dominant motivating factor behind their conduct.
4. That this concern could not have been adequately satisfied in a manner less restrictive of chiropractic competition.

In other words, all the AMA had to do to succeed in the second trial was to prove that it had been acting in good faith. Some degree of bias and hostility to chiropractic would not make its activities illegal. On the other side of the issue, to establish a case for injunctions that would prohibit the defendants from engaging in further antichiropractic behavior and violations of the Sherman Act, we the plaintiffs had to prove a continuing violation or a real threat of future violation—in other words, that an AMA conspiracy continued to exist or, if the conspiracy had technically been terminated, that the AMA had had no basic change of heart.

In the meantime, both the plaintiffs and the defendants prepared to petition the Supreme Court of the United States to hear the case. On April 30, 1984, we filed a petition with the Supreme Court to have certain of the guidelines for the retrial corrected or modified. As we had anticipated, the Supreme Court declined to hear the case. That sealed the decision that we would once again present our case, in a brand-new trial, before the U.S. District Court in the Northern District of Illinois.

*   *   *

On March 4, 1985, two months before we were scheduled to go back to court, the Illnois State Medical Society decided to settle with us.[14] This was a very welcome development. Apart from the American Medical Association, the Illinois State Medical Society was one of the largest medical organizations in America. Not only that, but it was located in the AMA's home state. They agreed to pay us $35,000 and to adopt a position rejecting any impediments (other than those existing in law) to cooperation between medical doctors and doctors of chiropractic. In exchange, we agreed not to sue them for any additional damages, attorneys' fees, or court costs.[15] We took the settlement as a sign that the ISMS knew we had a solid case and were likely to win. Psychologically, it gave us a great boost. The number of defendants was now down to eleven.

* * *

By the spring of 1987, our litigation had been in the works for over ten years, and the decision of the lower court was six and a half years behind us. It did not seem that long ago; the memories of what a disastrous trial it had been remained as fresh in our minds as if they had just occurred. All the things that had gone wrong in the courtroom were replayed in my mind whenever I thought about the trial. We could not know what the retrial would bring, and there were no assurances that another fiasco would be avoided.

In the first place, antitrust law is a complicated field, and if the next judge to hear our case was inexperienced with it, what assurance would we have that the same series of events would not take place a second time? The law is such an intricate thing. While lawyers specialize in the types of cases they argue, judges are not restricted in the types of cases they hear, and they need no special certification to preside over cases in specialized fields of the law. Without question, the defendants would try once again to bring in irrelevant material in an attempt to justify their past illegal conduct. Would the next judge repeat the mistake that had been made before and allow it as evidence? Would the defendants again paint such an outrageously inaccurate image of chiropractic that it would lead to another "not guilty" finding?

I had completely lost confidence in the jury system, at least as I saw it in practice. I had watched the jurors in the first trial be manipulated and misinformed, treated as if they were incapable of thinking for themselves. They had been spoon-fed a steady diet of information that they should not have heard in the first place and that was intended only to prejudice them, and they had not been allowed to hear other evidence that should have been permitted. The appeals court had described this problem well; it determined that the presence of a jury had allowed the real issues of the case to be submerged in what was later described as a "free-for-all between chiropractors and medical doctors, in which the scientific legitimacy of chiropractic was hotly debated and the comparative avarice of the adversaries was explored."[16]

I was convinced that we could ill afford another three-ring circus in the courtroom—a term that, to me, aptly described the histrionics that the lawyers had presented for the benefit of the jury, and that had ultimately obscured the basic question they were there to decide. For six and a half years, I had been considering pursuing a bench trial (a trial before a judge alone, without a jury) instead. The way to do this was to give up the right to sue for damages—in the case of antitrust law, treble damages (an award of money three times greater than your actual losses, designed to serve as punishment for the guilty party).

The more I thought about it, the more I liked this alternative. The main objective of our lawsuit, and the reason we had to win, was to destroy the boycott of chiropractic by the AMA and its allies. The truth had to be brought before the American people. The case had to be tried on the merit of the facts and the law. Imposing damages was not our purpose at all; this alone could not correct the situation. What good would all the money in the world be if the boycott continued to prevent the delivery of appropriate health care? Simply put, the boycott had to be stopped.

Yet there were risks involved in this option. If we had no right to monetary damages, the judge might decide that our case was moot and should be dismissed. George had told me there was approximately a 10-percent chance that this could happen. We had won the right to a retrial, and I hoped we would not jeopardize our chances of success if we chose to give up our claim for damages. Yet I knew there was no way I wanted to risk another disaster with a jury. Another jury trial would likely invite a replay of the AMA's theatrics during the first trial—after all, it had worked for them once.

I had never tried to tell the lawyers what to do or insisted on anything. This was going to be the one exception. I wasn't sure how George would react to this, and I hoped he would not be offended. To my relief, he wasn't. He considered that deciding to forego monetary damages could work to our advantage in the courtroom because it would make it plain that our primary interest was not one of money, but of principle. It would keep "the fictitious greed issue," as he put it, out of the proceedings, and that would help to keep the focus on antitrust, where it belonged. After we had discussed this at some length, George conferred with the other plaintiffs to weigh the pros and cons of the matter with them. And so it was decided: We would take our chances with the next judge, and hope that he would not throw out the case because we had waived our right to sue for damages.

Judge John A. Nordberg was assigned to our case. However, as the trial date drew closer, we learned that we would be getting a different judge, Susan Getzendanner. She had a reputation for being extremely intelligent, knowledgeable in the law, efficient, and fast. As the other judges in the district court were getting backlogged in cases, she was clearing out her docket and looking for work. She was planning to retire from the bench soon, but she was looking for some challenging cases to try before she did. While our case file was on the desk of Judge Nordberg, who had quite a backlog of cases, Judge Getzendanner happened to walk into his office and ask him if he had any interesting cases. He indicated the files on his desk, and she scanned through the cases. She noticed our case, was intrigued by it, and Judge Nordberg turned it over to her.

In doing our homework, trying to learn a little about the judge who would be trying our case, we found out that Judge Getzendanner had been the first woman to sit on the bench of the northern Illinois federal court. I heard from our legal team that the lawyers for the defense were quite unhappy that Judge Getzendanner had taken the case. No doubt her reputation as a brilliant, no-nonsense judge who was knowledgeable in matters of the law had reached their ears as well as our own. Although I did not yet have any firsthand information about this judge, whatever made the defendants' attorneys unhappy made me most happy indeed!

Of course, it was not that we were seeking preferential treatment, and we did not expect any from Judge Getzendanner. All we wanted was an honest and fair trial to decide on the issue of the antitrust violation, and we wanted it to be conducted flawlessly, so that it would pass the test of the appellate process. Regardless of who won, we knew that the ruling in the case would again be appealed to the Court of Appeals, and ultimately, again, to the United States Supreme Court. If the final decision was one that could withstand the appeals process, we felt confident enough that it would stand. If not, our problems would escalate. Financially, we could not afford a replay of what we had been through in 1980. The last reversal was costing us a great deal of money to retry, and while the American Medical Association seemed to have bottomless resources to spend on their legal defense, we were being stressed beyond the limit financially. This time, there could be no mistakes.

8

A REFRESHING RAIN

On May 5, 1987, we were back in court. There was a sense of déjà vu in being there; the scene was almost identical to that of the first trial. A different judge sat on the bench this time, but the same army of a dozen or more lawyers (minus those who had approached us for out-of-court settlements) filled the room, accompanied by junior lawyers and support staff. No jury had yet been selected, and the jury box remained empty.

George McAndrews approached the bench. With respect and style, he addressed the court, announcing that the plaintiffs were going to waive claims for damages and seek only injunctive relief—a court order to prevent the medical establishment from continuing its boycott of chiropractic. An obvious consequence of this waiver would be that the trial would be conducted without a jury.

You could have heard a pin drop in the courtroom. The gray and solemn faces of the defense lawyers appeared shocked by the unexpected announcement. Without a jury to influence, their entire strategy would need to be redrawn. There was no joy in their camp at a surprise like this.

Then followed a moment that was one of the most tense of the entire lawsuit. The possible effects of a bench trial, as opposed to a jury trial, must have been obvious to the defense lawyers. Would the defense move to have the suit dismissed? Would the judge rule in favor of it? Would she decide simply to dismiss the case on her own? For what seemed like an eternity, I sat there holding my breath, scarcely daring to move. My heart pounded so loudly within my chest it seemed to me that everyone sitting close to me must have heard it.

Finally, the judge spoke. "Now, Mr. McAndrews, look what you have gone and done!"

I wasn't sure if this remark meant that she was accepting the move for a bench trial or dismissing the case. But as Judge Getzendanner continued to speak, it gradually became clear to me that she was not going to dismiss the case, and that she would permit the bench trial. I breathed a heavy sigh of relief. We had survived one of the most critical moments of the retrial.

The Honorable Susan Getzendanner lived up to her reputation and proved to be absolutely brilliant in the courtroom. She had a gift for speed-reading and comprehension. As quickly as she turned the pages of the various exhibits, she could absorb and understand the documents' content, and she retained the information gleaned from them throughout the trial. It was an amazing thing to watch her in action.

Before long, it became evident that this was going to be an entirely different trial experience. Judge Getzendanner had a strong personality on the bench, and she was not going to tolerate the same theatrics we had seen during the first trial. The attorneys for the defense also appeared to realize this, and they could not have been too happy about it. But the other chiropractor-plaintiffs and I were thrilled with what we saw happening this time.

In the first trial, our case had not relied on expert opinions from medical physicians, and the case had become a matter of chiropractic doctors (the plaintiffs) versus medical doctors (the defendants). This time, our attorney determined to remedy this. He sought out the finest medical physicians in the country to testify as expert witnesses on our behalf. We wanted only world-class medical physicians who were held in the highest esteem by their peers. At the same time, to our benefit, new studies were being published all over the world offering substantial proof that chiropractic was not only a safe and effective method of treatment, but that it was clearly superior to medicine for certain musculoskeletal and neuromuscular problems.

We were fortunate enough to be able to obtain as evidence for our side testimony from John McMillan Mennell, M.D., who was known throughout the world as a leading medical orthopedist. In his long and illustrious career, he had authored numerous textbooks and an abundance of articles in medical journals, served as a professor at eight different medical schools in America, and visited many other medical schools as a guest speaker. His credentials were flawless. George used his testimony to establish the amount of training and expertise the typical M.D. had with the dynamics of the musculoskeletal system. George read from a transcript of testimony Dr. Mennell had given in 1980, under questioning from an attorney for the AMA. The professor made a startling revelation.

The AMA's attorney asked, "I think you [said that medical residents receive] four or five hours of training in manipulative therapy—is this correct?"

Dr. Mennell replied, "I think I said zero hours, didn't I, for the most part?"

Apparently finding Dr. Mennell's response hard to believe, the AMA lawyer pressed him further. "What I'm trying to determine is, when you talk about zero hours' training in manipulation, what particular definition of 'manipulation' were you referring to?"

Dr. Mennell answered, "I think my testimony was that if you ask a bunch of new residents who come into a hospital for the first time how long they spent in studying the problems of the musculoskeletal system, they would, for the most part, reply, 'Zero to about four hours.' I think that was my testimony."

The attorney asked, "The musculoskeletal system comprises what portion of the body?"

"As a system, about 60 percent of the body."

"Is your testimony," the AMA attorney asked, "that the residents to whom you just referred told you they had no training whatsoever relating to problems as to 60 percent of the body?"

Dr. Mennell replied, "That is just about right."

Once again, the AMA's lawyer seemed to be astonished at Dr. Mennell's testimony. "Is it your testimony that it is your understanding that the entire medical school curriculum is devoted to about 40 percent of the body?"

Without hesitation, Dr. Mennell answered, "Yes, sir."[1]

Dr. Mennell's testimony caught the attorneys for the defense off guard. It also served to explain why medical doctors simply do not have the comprehensive understanding of the musculoskeletal system that chiropractors have. His testimony beautifully illustrated the need for interprofessional cooperation. Each health care profession has its domain of expertise, and in order to maximize health care in America, each must be permitted to contribute where it can offer the optimum benefit to patients.

Our attorney called as a witness a prominent orthopedic surgeon and radiologist, Per Freitag, M.D., from Des Plaines, Illinois. Dr. Freitag was a professor of orthopedic surgery at Northwestern University and had a Ph.D. in anatomy.

Under oath in the courtroom, Dr. Freitag explained a study he had conducted comparing John F. Kennedy Hospital (now Our Lady of Resurrection) in Chicago with Lutheran General Hospital in Park Ridge, Illinois. These two hospitals were located about half an hour's drive apart from each other and served patients from essentially the same kind of community. JFK Hospital had initiated a chiropractic department, and was allowing chiropractors to treat patients with low back pain who were in the orthopedic ward of the hospital. Lutheran General had no such program. Since Dr. Freitag was on the staff of both hospitals, he could conduct a comparison study on the efficacy of chiropractic in hospitals. He testified under oath as to his conclusion: The average hospital stay of orthopedic patients was cut in half when they received in-hospital chiropractic care concurrently with other medical treatment.

George asked him, "Are you interested in getting these patients better faster?"

Dr. Freitag replied, "Absolutely."

"For how long a period of time have you been caring for patients at Lutheran General?" George questioned.

"Since the summer of 1978."

George continued, "For how long a period of time have you been caring for patients at JFK?"

"Since May of last year," Dr. Freitag answered.

"Can you tell us," George asked, "in your experience, at which hospital you are able to get your patients better faster?"

With no hesitation, Dr. Freitag said, "At the John F. Kennedy."

George probed, "Have you been able to reach a conclusion as to the reason for that?"

Dr. Freitag was firm in his response. "The only difference

that I can see is that the patients at John F. Kennedy get chiropractic manipulations. And in my experience, the patients at
JFK, almost without fail, get out of the hospital in a week, six,
seven days. At Lutheran, it usually takes, oh, not uncommonly
fourteen days."

"Is that—is it a benefit to the patient in your experience to be
able to get them out of the hospital quicker?"

"Absolutely," Dr. Freitag testified.[2]

Other studies were similarly reviewed during the trial. Two
independent studies were presented as evidence that chiropractic care was able to get people back to work in half the time and
at half the cost of medical care. One of these was a 1971 report
by Rolland A. Martin, M.D., medical director for the Oregon
Workmen's Compensation Board.[3] He had examined records
from 1971 of industrial injuries to workers, and concluded that
chiropractic care had a 2-to-1 advantage over other types of
conservative therapy in time loss back-injury claims; chiropractic got injured workers back on the job in half the time and at
half the cost of medical therapy.[4] The second was a 1975 report
published by C. Richard Wolf, M.D., on a study of 629 comparable injuries found in workers' compensation claims in California
during 1972.[5] Dr. Wolf concluded that doctors of chiropractic
(D.C.s) were twice as effective as M.D.s at treating comparable
injuries, at every level of severity, measured in terms of how fast
they enabled injured workers to return to work.[6] (For an abstract
of these studies, *see* Appendix I.)

* * *

At the first trial, six and a half years earlier, we had attempted
to bring H. Doyl Taylor into court, but his son had insisted he
was too ill to come to Chicago to testify, and our efforts were
unsuccessful. We now decided to make another attempt. Taylor
had been the director of the AMA's Department of Investigation,
and also had been acting secretary of the AMA's Committee on
Quackery, the committee devoted to the elimination of chiropractic. Once again, Taylor insisted he was not healthy enough
to make the trip to Chicago, so our attorney got permission to go
to Arizona and videotape his testimony, which would then be
brought back to Chicago for the court to see.

Taylor then insisted that he was too ill to testify at all. Judge Getzendanner issued a court order mandating that the AMA have Taylor submit to physical examination to evaluate whether or not he truly was unable to testify. Having either a medical doctor or a chiropractor do the examination might have been construed as introducing bias, so Taylor was examined by an osteopath, who pronounced him to be in excellent health, and most certainly able to testify on videotape. With the osteopath's report in hand, Judge Getzendanner remarked, "That man is healthy enough to *walk* to Chicago!" George McAndrews then flew to Arizona, along with several of the defendants' attorneys, to take videotapes of Taylor's testimony.

For eleven years, as secretary of the Committee on Quackery, Doyl Taylor had repeatedly confirmed that it was the AMA's objective to completely eliminate the chiropractic profession. Now, under oath on videotape, Taylor denied that his committee had been working for the elimination of chiropractic, maintaining instead that it had only been concerned that chiropractic was a health hazard.

During the course of questioning, Taylor made a startling admission. He said that when he took the position with the AMA, he did not "know a chiropractor from an antelope," and that even all these years later, he had only a "vague" idea of what chiropractors did. Apparently he had been laboring for years to eliminate a form of health care he did not even understand. But perhaps the single most revealing moment during Taylor's videotaped deposition occurred when he was asked if he knew that there were Ph.D.s teaching in accredited chiropractic colleges. He acknowledged that he did, but then sneered that they were all of various ethnic minority backgrounds.[7] I couldn't help wondering whether this display of bigotry and contempt was a reflection of the mentality of Taylor's former masters. Did the AMA representatives in the room see it, too? Were they shamed by it? Or were they blind to it?

* * *

During the second trial, an interesting and crucial document surfaced. This was a letter that had been sent by Irvin Hendryson, M.D., an orthopedic surgeon and AMA trustee, to

Robert Throckmorton, the association's general counsel.[8] In this letter, Dr. Hendryson reported on what was very possibly the first controlled trial of orthopedic versus chiropractic care. This was a study conducted in a military orthopedic ward during World War II.

Dr. Hendryson's letter reported on a clinical comparison of two groups of enlisted military servicemen who were treated for low back pain. One group was treated with chiropractic adjustments; the other was a control group that received standard medical treatment. The United States Army provided Dr. Hendryson with an ideal environment for patient control. The study showed that chiropractic had impressive successes with some cases in which medical treatment had failed. The chiropractic adjustments were at least as effective as some of the best medical treatments; therefore, Dr. Hendryson suggested, chiropractic should be made available in all hospital orthopedic wards. Dr. Hendryson further noted that after the war, at the University of Colorado, he had observed that chiropractic adjustments were very helpful to women in the third trimester of pregnancy. He said that women were able to carry and deliver their children with less discomfort if they received chiropractic adjustments.*[9]

The Hendryson letter proved beyond any doubt that the AMA and its Committee on Quackery had known all along that chiropractic was effective. While there had been many studies over the years that had shown this (*see* Appendix I, A Partial List of Studies on Chiropractic), this particular letter, reporting on findings over forty years old, had been sent by one of the organization's own trustees to its general counsel. This made clear what the AMA did not want the public to know—that chiropractic provided an ideal health care alternative in areas where medi-

---

*As this evidence was revealed, one of the attorneys for the defense fairly sneered at the idea that a woman who had received chiropractic adjustments might have an easier time during childbirth. At this, Judge Getzendanner looked up and pointed at him, her index finger wagging slowly from side to side like a metronome, and cut him short. Dryly, she reminded him that *he* had never had to give birth. (The judge herself was the mother of two children.) The defense counsel, apparently realizing that his derisive attitude was probably a major error in judgment, promptly sat down and shut up.

cine had failed, *and* that the AMA knew this.[10] The latter point
was important, because the "patient care defense" the AMA was
putting forth rested on the premise that the organization's sole,
true motive in boycotting chiropractic was concern for the welfare of patients. For this to be valid, the AMA had to demonstrate
that it was objectively reasonable for them to believe that chiropractic manipulation was useless if not downright harmful. The
existence of the Hendryson letter proved that this could not have
been the case.

Equally noteworthy was the fact that the committee was
made aware of the fact that some medical physicians believed
that chiropractic was effective. Furthermore, evidence presented in the courtroom revealed that in the course of their
lengthy boycott, the members of the Committee on Quackery
had become fully aware that there was no objectively reasonable concern sufficient to justify a boycott of the entire chiropractic profession.[11]

* * *

During the trial, the defense attorneys never acknowledged
that anything the AMA had ever done had been wrong. Much
of their attention was focused on the claim that *if* there had
ever been a boycott of chiropractic, it had ended in 1980, when
the AMA adopted its new ethical standards (*see* The AMA
Reverses Itself . . . Or Does It?, page 89). For the plaintiffs,
George McAndrews countered with proof from the AMA's
own files—documents proclaiming the boycott's earlier success. The memo of January 4, 1971, from the AMA's Committee on Quackery to the AMA Board of Trustees was evidence
that the AMA had considered its boycott successful—that is,
that it was achieving the goal of containing chiropractic, and
that the ultimate elimination of chiropractic well underway
(see page 45).[12] George further argued that since the AMA
revised its ethical code to eliminate the prohibition on cooperating with chiropractors, chiropractors had been seeing an
increase in the demand for their services and, consequently, a
growth in their professional incomes, which further verified
the earlier success of the boycott. He also argued that because
the AMA had never explicitly stated, in writing, that medical

doctors could now ethically consult with chiropractors, the boycott had in effect continued.*

In their arguments, the defendants' attorneys now asserted that it was in fact the antichiropractic criticism and conduct of their clients that had stimulated the chiropractic's remarkable growth, the improvement in its public image, and the many advances it had made in the six and a half years that had passed since the first trial began. To bolster this claim, they brought in an economist named William Lynk, who argued that the AMA's conduct actually *encouraged* competition, by means of a mechanism he called "nonverbal communication."[13] The defendants were now trying to take credit for improvements in chiropractic! I thought I had heard just about

---

*Actually, a case that could have proved that the boycott continued was then taking place just west of Chicago in the town of Elmhurst, Illinois, where a chiropractor and a medical neurologist had joined forces in a practice they called a "neuro-spinal center." They referred patients to each other, consulted together, and shared space at their respective offices. The neurologist's office was in a condominium in a professional center that also housed a number of other medical offices. The doctors who occupied those offices began to put pressure on the neurologist to terminate his association with the chiropractor. The neurologist received a notice from the president of the condominium owners association advising him that he was in violation of his ownership agreement and that he must immediately cease using his condominium unit for any activity related to chiropractic services. The other M.D.s cut off their own referrals to the neurologist, his hospital staff privileges were suspended, and a surgical audit of his practice was initiated. As a result of these and other pressure tactics, the neurologist was forced to break off his business relationship with the chiropractor. Unfortunately, we learned about this case too late to use it in court, but the chiropractor later filed his own lawsuit against the doctors, the hospital, and the condominium association that had forced an end to his relationship with the neurologist. The suit was based on the federal Racketeer and Corrupt Organizations (RICO) Act, originally enacted as a weapon against organized crime. It charged the defendants with engaging in a pattern of racketeering activity involving threats that met the legal definition of extortion, and the court upheld the chiropractor's right to sue on this basis. Whether the defendants in this case would have been convicted we do not know, because the parties ultimately reached a settlement and the neurologist and chiropractor were able to resume their professional association. But it did serve to establish another possible approach to fighting the illegal antichiropractic boycott.

everything there was to hear in the way of rationalization for the AMA's conduct, but this was certainly a novel twist.

There is an ancient Chinese proverb that says a gem cannot be polished without friction, and neither is a man perfected without trials. There was no doubt in my mind that chiropractic was arising from all of its adversities as a brilliant gem among the health care professions. But to give the American Medical Association the credit for this? Next they would be sending us a bill for their assistance in helping chiropractic succeed as a profession!

This line of reasoning threw all of us off guard. It was preposterous. But how could a claim like this be put into proper perspective? How in the world does an attorney respond to such a thing? When George left the courtroom that evening, he was pondering the AMA's new line of defense.

When the court was called to order the next morning, George was the first to address the court. He had the perfect answer to the AMA's new approach. Slowly, he spoke of the AMA's new justification for its behavior—and then said that it reminded him of a German U-boat commander saying he was responsible for the performance of American Olympic swimmers because by sinking their ships, he had taught them to swim. His point was well made, and it brought a loud guffaw from the judge and laughter throughout the courtroom—including from some of the lawyers for the defense. After that day, the defendants never again tried to take the credit for the tremendous growth of chiropractic.

* * *

I was called to the witness stand on the afternoon of Thursday, May 21, 1987. The defendants knew that chiropractic was begun by Dr. Daniel David Palmer after he corrected the hearing of a deaf janitor. They apparently hoped to make me—and chiropractic—appear foolish by inducing me to suggest that hearing could be affected by adjustment of the spine. I was questioned regarding what I knew about modern research on improvements in hearing brought about by chiropractic adjustments.

Actually, such a case had been corroborated by the Royal Commission of Inquiry on Chiropractic in New Zealand.[14] This case involved a young deaf girl whose parents had taken her to see an ear, nose, and throat specialist. He recommended surgery, which they were reluctant to agree to. Since the mother had been successfully treated for a back ailment by a chiropractor, she decided to take her daughter to the chiropractor, who adjusted the girl's spine in the area below her neck. The following morning, her hearing began to improve. When the same ear, nose, and throat specialist reexamined her hearing, he found it had improved to a level of 100/98 (meaning that she could hear at 98 feet what a normal person can hear at 100). The M.D. warned the child's parents that the improvement was only temporary, and that they would be back to see him in six months, but he was wrong; the girl retained her hearing.[15] There have also been other substantiated reports of chiropractic adjustment as a successful treatment for hearing impairment.

The defendants' cross-examination of me went on to consider chiropractic office practices, my use of x-rays, and my attendance at "practice management" seminars.[16] The opposing attorneys' questions seemed designed to imply that I was guilty of questionable practices, but without allowing me to give the full story. Later, in redirect examination, George gave me an opportunity to set the record straight. The defense lawyers had attempted to say that chiropractors insisted on performing maintenance treatments—adjustments used to keep the spine in alignment, rather than to relieve specific symptoms—and that this proved we were more interested in making money than in serving our patients.

"Dr. Wilk," he asked, "have you ever forced anyone to have a maintenance adjustment?"

"Never," I told him firmly.

"Okay," he pressed, "how does a maintenance adjustment come about?"

"Initially, a patient will come in with a history of having problems," I explained, "and upon receiving adjustments and getting their health restored, we give them the option that now that they are feeling better, particularly if they have a chronic history of many years' duration, to come in periodically, just as a maintenance tune-up, somewhat like you bring your car in for an occasional oil change. You don't wait until the motor burns out before you do repairs."

George asked, "Is the option left up to the patient to return?"

"Oh, yes," I replied.

"All right," George continued, "and is it the patient's option to stay away from you and not give you any money for those [maintenance adjustments]?"

"Naturally," I nodded. "Of course, sure."[17]

George also asked me why I felt I needed the cooperative services of a hospital.

"Let's take a hypothetical situation," I said. "A person is involved in an automobile accident. His wife is thrown through the window and killed. He, in the process, received lacerations. And in a place like this, the driver of the car who felt responsible may need psychiatric help. He may need a surgeon to repair the cuts. He may need an internist for any possible internal bleeding. He also needs a chiropractor for the mechanical structural injury he may have. And this [a hospital] would provide an ideal setting [for treatment] through cooperative efforts."

I concluded that a chiropractor practicing in a hospital—which was impossible as long as the illegal boycott was in force—would be able to provide the structural manipulative portion of the treatment, while other physicians attended to the other aspects of treatment. If health care professionals were able to cooperate in this way, I emphasized, patients would be able to receive the full range of necessary therapies instead of partial care.[18]

Changing directions again, George asked, "Did you ever criticize the Parker seminars?" These were the seminars designed to teach chiropractors about different aspects of the profession, especially the business side of running a practice (see page 69). It was at a Parker seminar in 1976 that I had arranged for Sore Throat to tell thousands of chiropractors what he knew about the AMA's activities against their profession, in the hope of enlisting their support for legal action against the organization.

"Yes, I have."

"Can you tell us how you criticized it?"

"This had to have been about seventeen or eighteen years ago [when I attended the Parker seminar]. At the end of the Parker seminar, Parker would pass out a slip of paper to every chiropractor in the room, and of course, if they had some very positive comments, he would publish them in his publication. Mine was critical of some of the selling promotional aspects of it and, of course, he never published that."

"Dr. Wilk," George continued, "you stated that there was a large portion of the Parker seminars that you thought had value?"

"Yes. He had many technique seminars given by different chiropractors. He had x-ray seminars that represented a large percent of his program. He had seminars on diseases, seminars—it was almost like a postgraduate course, if you look at these seminars."

"Did he bring in experts from around the country?"

"Indeed he did."

"Were some of those medical physicians?"

"M.D.s, very prominent names that everyone would instantly recognize."

"I believe [one of your answers in a deposition was] that it was a survivalist course. What did you mean by that?"

"What I meant is that due to the boycott and the fact that the chiropractors were struggling to survive because of the containment and elimination committee of the American Medical Association, many of the chiropractors were suffering with an image concept. They felt depressed. They felt put down. They felt isolated, and it gave them a chance to get together and exchange ideas, break bread, and build up their . . . self-image and confidence in themselves through association with other successful people, and especially with prominent medical [and] osteopathic educators who they could identify with and feel good about themselves."

"I have no further questions," George said, and we were finished.[19] We had touched on several aspects of chiropractic that had come under fire from the defense attorneys, and I felt I had responded to them in such a way that I gave clear proof that current practices in the field were not only effective in treatment, but also were safe and prudent, and provided a superior health care service.

The other plaintiffs followed me on the witness stand. Their testimony was essentially a recapitulation of what they had said during the previous trial.

* * *

Initially, Judge Getzendanner had not planned to allow any chiropractic patients to testify as to the effectiveness of the treatment they had received. She felt it was not relevant to an antitrust lawsuit, since the effectiveness of chiropractic was not at issue; the attempted restraint of trade was. However, because the defendants insisted that medicine and chiropractic were not in competition with each other, she decided to allow some patients to testify so as to establish whether or not there was in fact competition between the professions.

It was a pleasure to have a couple of my patients brought in as witnesses. One such person was a woman named Sharon, whose husband, Joe, had been a patient of mine for some time. Sharon suffered from persistent headaches, and for eighteen months had never been free of pain. She had spent thousands of dollars seeking help from medical doctors, but with minimal—indeed, insignificant—results. Her husband had urged her, over that long period of time, to try chiropractic adjustments, but she did not believe chiropractic could help her when neither the finest medical doctors in Chicago nor a famous headache clinic had helped.

"Try it," her husband would say. "What have you got to lose?" But she resisted.

One day, they told me, Sharon had said to Joe, "I wish I was a horse!"

Joe responded, "Why in the world would you say that?"

"Well, because if I was a horse, you could shoot me!"

Joe became impatient. "I'm telling you, Sharon," he said, "don't be so damned stubborn! Go to my chiropractor!"

Finally, in October 1986, she broke down and decided to come in for treatment, just to put an end to her husband's persistent urging. She received one adjustment, and immediately noted an improvement. After her second adjustment, the pain was completely gone, and she had never had the headaches again. Sharon related her experience under oath for the court record.

* * *

The American Hospital Association (AHA) settled with us on June 12, 1987. The trial was proceeding and appeared to be drawing to a close. Perhaps the AHA lawyers felt it was time to cut their losses. The terms of the settlement with that organization satisfied one of the major goals of the lawsuit: It gave us a legally binding agreement that there would be no further impediments to chiropractors practicing in hospitals. The agree-

ment specified in a policy statement, which was not to be re-
tracted for at least ten years, that individual hospitals should be
free to determine their own policies on offering chiropractic
services in a hospital setting. It further indicated that the AHA
had:

> no objection to a hospital granting privileges to doctors of chiroprac-
> tic for the purposes of (1) administering chiropractic treatment . . . ;
> (2) furthering the clinical education and training of doctors of chiro-
> practic; or (3) having . . . x-rays, clinical laboratory tests and reports
> thereon made for doctors of chiropractic and their patients and/or
> previously taken x-rays, clinical laboratory tests and reports made
> available to them by [hospital medical staff and consultants] upon
> the authorization of the patient involved.[20]

Finally, the policy statement said that individual hospitals'
decisions as to whether they wished to employ or otherwise
professionally associate with chiropractors should be made on
grounds "no different [than] with other licensed health care
professionals," and that the AHA "specifically disavows any
unlawful effort . . . to undermine the public's confidence in the
profession of chiropractic."[21]

* * *

The trial came to an end on July 2. Once again, it was time to return
home and wait—and to hope and pray that this time, the decision
would be in our favor. Finally, on August 27, 1987, District Judge
Susan Getzendanner, in her final case before retiring from the
bench, passed down her 101-page decision. The principal defendants remaining—the American Medical Association, the American College of Radiology, the American College of Surgeons, and
the American Academy of Orthopaedic Surgeons—were found
guilty, as alleged, of joining a conspiracy against chiropractors in
violation of antitrust law. Judge Getzendanner ruled that:

> [The AMA and its leaders had] instituted a boycott of chiroprac-
> tors in the mid-1960s by informing AMA members that chiroprac-
> tors were unscientific practitioners and that it was unethical for
> a medical physician to associate with chiropractors. The purpose
> of the boycott was to contain and eliminate the chiropractic
> profession. This conduct constituted a conspiracy among the

AMA and its members and an unreasonable restraint of trade in violation of Section 1 of the Sherman Act.[22]

The precise form of the court orders would follow. The cases against two of the defendants, the Joint Commission on Accreditation of Hospitals and the American College of Physicians, were dismissed.

On September 24, 1987, after Judge Getzendanner had passed down her guilty verdict and before she issued the permanent injunction ordering the defendants to change their behavior with respect to chiropractic, the American College of Radiology (ACR) settled with us. As a result of the financial settlement of $200,000, every radiologist who was a member of the ACR received an individual assessment to fund the legal fees (each one was required to pay $100).[23] The radiologists had been particularly antagonistic toward chiropractic, and had fought very hard in the lawsuit. Indeed, they stood to lose a great deal economically. Since the boycott had prohibited radiologists from providing chiropractors with x-ray services for their patients, most chiropractors had had no other choice but to purchase their own costly x-ray equipment. Consequently, in many small towns, where there were no hospitals to provide radiology services, if limitations on cooperation between chiropractors and medical doctors were removed, patients would be able to get x-rays from a local chiropractor, instead of having to travel to distant hospital radiology departments. Thus, conveniently located chiropractors could potentially take business away from radiologists. This was a serious competitive threat, and the radiologists fought it until the last reasonable moment. I am sure that after the judgment against them, they felt it was simply not worth resisting any longer, and concluded that paying additional legal fees to wait another three years or so for a ruling from the Court of Appeals, just to get a chance at yet another trial, would not be worth it.

Professionally speaking, this was a landmark settlement. At the time of the trial, the ACR had been the only defendant with an open policy against cooperation with the chiropractic profession. As part of the settlement, the ACR adopted and published a policy statement that was to remain in force for at least ten years and that stipulated:

There are and should be no ethical or collective impediments to inter-professional association and cooperation between doctors of chiropractic and medical radiologists in any setting where such association may occur. . . . [Radiologists] are urged to be sensitive to and consider the legitimate radiologic needs of all licensed members of the healing arts, including doctors of chiropractic.[24]

The American College of Surgeons (ACS) also settled with us on September 24, 1987. This settlement required the adoption and publication of a policy, not to be altered for at least five years, preventing the institution of ethical or collective restraints on full professional cooperation between doctors of chiropractic and medical physicians, and stipulating that such cooperation might include referrals, group practice arrangements, participation by M.D.s and D.C.s in all health care delivery systems, treatment and services by chiropractors in and through hospitals, and participation in student exchange programs and education programs.[25]

The terms of the ACS settlement also included a payment of $200,000 to the Kentuckiana Children's Center, a nonprofit hospital founded by Lorraine Golden, D.C., that provided free services and care to handicapped children.[26] This was a particularly happy postscript to the trial (*see* The Boycott of Kentuckiana, page 170).

Also after the guilty verdict, the American Academy of Orthopaedic Surgeons decided to settle with us.[27] The individual defendants—Doyl Taylor, Joseph Sabatier, Thomas Ballantine, and James Sammons—had all retired by this time, and they had been dropped from the suit. This left the AMA as the sole defendant.

Judge Getzendanner's court orders, issued on September 27, 1987, included an injunction forbidding the AMA to engage in any collective boycott against chiropractors, and forcing the AMA to tell its members that the organization's official position now was that it was ethical for medical doctors to associate professionally with chiropractors.[28] (For the full text of the injunction, see page 173.) An injunction is a court order that prohibits a party from engaging in certain actions; the court may issue an injunction when there is a recognized threat that a party's illegal conduct may recur. In the case of the AMA, the court found such injunctive relief appropriate. The court's order concerning the AMA specified the following:

The Boycott of Kentuckiana

The AMA's illegal boycott of chiropractic had far-reaching nega-
tive effects nationwide. One of the saddest examples concerned a
center for developmentally disabled children located near Louis-
ville, Kentucky. The Kentuckiana Center for Education, Health,
and Research (originally the Kentuckiana Children's Chiroprac-
tic Center) was founded in 1955 by Dr. Lorraine Golden, a
chiropractor who is affectionately viewed by many as the "Mother
Teresa of the chiropractic profession." Dr. Golden was able to
obtain an unoccupied twelve-acre army hospital site and there
founded a private nonprofit, nonsectarian organization that pro-
vided free medical care—including physical therapy, psychologi-
cal counseling, chiropractic care, speech therapy, and referrals for
medical, surgical, dental, and optometric care—to handicapped
children. The property was later given to Dr. Golden by the
government.

Over the years, Dr. Golden was supported by local civic, labor,
and religious groups who recognized her compassion and dedica-
tion. They conducted fund drives and did volunteer work for
Kentuckiana. Dr. Golden applied also for federal grant money and
approached many of the better known national charitable funding
organizations, but these consistently turned her down. Un-
daunted, she persevered, often with very limited funds, and
somehow she managed to provide millions of dollars' worth of free
care to thousands of children over the course of forty years.

One of the greatest obstacles she faced was the effort by the
Kentucky Medical Society and the local Jefferson County Medical
Society to isolate Kentuckiana by preventing physicians from
working there and by attempting to obstruct charitable funding.[1]
The Jefferson County Medical Society even went so far as to adopt
a resolution condemning the center.[2] Dr. Golden was made to
understand that this opposition might cease if only she would
eliminate chiropractic from her program, but she refused, main-
taining that neither chiropractic nor medicine was sufficient by
itself, nor was one discipline superior to the other.

During the trial, Dr. Golden had a chance to come in to court as a witness. She spoke of how a pediatrician had been told by the local medical society that she should not associate professionally with the center because of the chiropractic care provided there. This forced the doctor to stop visiting the children's center, lest she face serious repercussions. Instead, the center had to load the children into an unmarked van and, under cover of night, drive the children twelve miles to the doctor's office for medical care.[3] As Judge Getzendanner listened to the testimony, she looked very grim and took profuse notes.

The fact that Kentuckiana ultimately received $200,000 as a result of the trial was particularly welcome to us, and it couldn't have come at a better time. On August 15, 1987, the Urban Renewal and Community Development Agency of Louisville had sold Kentuckiana nineteen acres of land adjoining the children's center. Though the land was valued at $800,000, the agency sold it for only one dollar, on the condition that Kentuckiana succeeded in raising sufficient funds to construct facilities for the care of up to 1,000 special children. Announcement of the $200,000 settlement came just one month later.

1. That the AMA had to print the full text of the injunction in its own publication, the *Journal of the American Medical Association (JAMA)*.

2. That the AMA had to send via first-class mail a letter to each of its 280,000 members informing them of the injunction.

3. That the AMA had to modify its written ethics opinions to remove chiropractors from the "unscientific practitioners" section; and they had to have a subtitle designated "chiropractors" or "chiropractic" that would carry an instruction that it is ethical for medical physicians to associate with chiropractors whenever, in their judgment, it would benefit the patient to do so.[29]

In one respect, the situation now was similar to that of six and a half years before, only this time, we were in the driver's seat;

the court had found in our favor. But the matter really wasn't settled yet. The final battle would take place in the U.S. Court of Appeals. The American Medical Association, the only group among the defendants judged guilty who had not reached a settlement with us, had the right to take the decision back to the appellate court to plead once again for a new trial. So once again, we waited.

Text of the Court Order in *Wilk* v. *AMA*

The following is the full text of the court order issued on September 26, 1987, by Judge Susan Getzendanner against the American Medical Association:

The court conducted a lengthy trial of this case in May and June of 1987 and on August 27, 1987, issued a 101-page opinion finding that the American Medical Association ("AMA") and its members participated in a conspiracy against chiropractors in violation of the nation's antitrust laws. Thereafter an opinion dated September 25, 1987, was substituted for the August 27, 1987, opinion. The question now before the court is the form of injunctive relief that the court will order.

As part of the injunctive relief to be ordered by the court against the AMA, the AMA shall be required to send a copy of this Permanent Injunction Order to each of its current members. The members of the AMA are bound by the terms of the Permanent Injunction Order if they act in concert with the AMA to violate the terms of the order. Accordingly, it is important that the AMA members understand the order and the reasons why the order has been entered.

The AMA's Boycott and Conspiracy

In the early 1960s, the AMA decided to contain and eliminate chiropractic as a profession. In 1963 the AMA's Committee on Quackery was formed. The committee worked aggressively—both overtly and covertly—to eliminate chiropractic. One of the principal means used by the AMA to achieve its goal was to make it unethical for medical physicians to professionally associate with chiropractors. Under Principle 3 of the AMA's Principles of Medical Ethics, it was unethical for a physician to associate with an "unscientific practitioner," and in 1966 the AMA's House of Delegates passed a resolution calling chiropractic an unscientific cult. To complete the circle, in 1967 the AMA's Judicial Council issued an opinion under Principle 3 holding that it was unethical for a physician to associate professionally with chiropractors.

The AMA's purpose was to prevent medical physicians from refer-
ring patients to chiropractors and accepting referrals of patients from
chiropractors, to prevent chiropractors from obtaining access to hospital
diagnostic services and membership on hospital medical staffs, to pre-
vent medical physicians from teaching at chiropractic colleges or engag-
ing in any joint research, and to prevent any cooperation between the
two groups in the delivery of health care services.

The AMA believed that the boycott worked—that chiropractic
would have achieved greater gains in the absence of the boycott. Since
no medical physician would want to be considered unethical by his
peers, the success of the boycott is not surprising. However, chiro-
practic achieved licensing in all 50 states during the existence of the
Committee on Quackery.

The Committee on Quackery was disbanded in 1975 and some of the
committee's activities became publicly known. Several lawsuits were
filed by or on behalf of chiropractors and this case was filed in 1976.

Change in AMA Position on Chiropractic

In 1977, the AMA began to change its position on chiropractic. The
AMA's Judicial Council adopted new opinions under which medical
physicians could refer patients to chiropractors, but there was still the
proviso that the medical physician should be confident that the services
to be provided on referral would be performed in accordance with
accepted scientific standards. In 1979, the AMA's House of Delegates
adopted Report UU which said that not everything that a chiropractor
may do is without therapeutic value, but it stopped short of saying that
such things were based on scientific standards. It was not until 1980
that the AMA revised its Principles of Medical Ethics to eliminate
Principle 3. Until Principle 3 was formally eliminated, there was
considerable ambiguity about the AMA's position. The ethics code
adopted in 1980 provided that a medical physician "shall be free to
choose whom to serve, with whom to associate, and the environment in
which to provide medical services."

The AMA settled three chiropractic lawsuits by stipulating and
agreeing that under the current opinions of the Judicial Council a
physician may, without fear of discipline or sanction by the AMA, refer

a patient to a duly licensed chiropractor when he believes that referral may benefit the patient. The AMA confirmed that a physician may also choose to accept or to decline patients sent to him by a duly licensed chiropractor. Finally, the AMA confirmed that a physician may teach at a chiropractic college or seminar. These settlements were entered into in 1978, 1980, and 1986.

The AMA's present position on chiropractic, as stated to the court, is that it is ethical for a medical physician to professionally associate with chiropractors provided the physician believes that such association is in the best interest of his patient. This position has not previously been communicated by the AMA to its members.

Antitrust Laws

Under the Sherman Act, every combination or conspiracy in restraint of trade is illegal. The court has held that the conduct of the AMA and its members constituted a conspiracy in restraint of trade based on the following facts: the purpose of the boycott was to eliminate chiropractic; chiropractors are in competition with some medical physicians; the boycott had substantial anti-competitive effects; there were no pro-competitive effects of the boycott; and the plaintiffs were injured as a result of the conduct. These facts add up to a violation of the Sherman Act.

In this case, however, the court allowed the defendants the opportunity to establish a "patient care defense" which has the following elements:
(1) that they genuinely entertained a concern for what they perceive as scientific method in the care of each person with whom they have entered into a doctor-patient relationship; (2) that this concern is objectively reasonable; (3) that this concern has been the dominant motivating factor in the defendants' promulgation of Principle 3 and in the conduct intended to implement it; and (4) that this concern for scientific method in patient care could not have been adequately satisfied in a manner less restrictive of competition.

The court concluded that the AMA had a genuine concern for scientific methods in patient care, and that this concern was the dominant factor motivating the AMA's conduct. However, the AMA *failed to establish that throughout the entire period of the boycott, from 1966 to 1980, this concern was objectively reasonable. The court reached that conclusion on the basis of extensive testimony from both witnesses for the plaintiffs and the AMA that some forms of chiropractic treatment are effective and the fact that the AMA recognized that chiropractic began to change in the early 1970s. Since the boycott was not formally over until Principle 3 was eliminated in 1980, the court found that the AMA was unable to establish that during the entire period of the conspiracy its position was objectively reasonable. Finally, the court ruled that the AMA's concern for scientific method in patient care could have been adequately satisfied in a manner less restrictive of competition and that a nationwide conspiracy to eliminate a licensed profession was not justified by the concern for scientific method. On the basis of these findings, the court concluded that the AMA had failed to establish the patient care defense.*

None of the court's findings constituted a judicial endorsement of chiropractic. All of the parties to the case, including the plaintiffs and the AMA, agreed that chiropractic treatment of diseases such as diabetes, high blood pressure, cancer, heart disease and infectious disease is not proper, and that the historic theory of chiropractic, that there is a single cause and cure of disease, was wrong. There was disagreement between the parties as to whether chiropractors should engage in diagnosis. There was evidence that the chiropractic theory of subluxations was unscientific, and evidence that some chiropractors engaged in unscientific practices. The court did not reach the question of whether chiropractic theory was in fact scientific. However, the evidence in the case was that some forms of chiropractic manipulation of the spine and joints was therapeutic. AMA witnesses, including the present Chairman of the Board of Trustees of the AMA, testified that some forms of treatment by chiropractors, including manipulation, can be therapeutic in the treatment of conditions such as back pain syndrome.

Need for Injunctive Relief

Although the conspiracy ended in 1980, there are lingering effects of the illegal boycott and conspiracy which require an injunction. Some medical physicians' individual decisions on whether or not to professionally associate with chiropractors are still affected by the boycott. The injury to chiropractors' reputations which resulted from the boycott has not been repaired. Chiropractors suffer current economic injury as a result of the boycott. The AMA has never affirmatively acknowledged that there are and should be no collective impediments to professional association and cooperation between chiropractors and medical physicians, except as provided by law. Instead, the AMA has consistently argued that its conduct has not violated the antitrust laws.

Most importantly, the court believes that it is important that the AMA members be made aware of the present AMA position that it is ethical for a medical physician to professionally associate with a chiropractor if the physician believes it is in the best interest of his patient, so that the lingering effects of the illegal group boycott against chiropractors finally can be dissipated.

Under the law, every medical physician, institution, and hospital has the right to make an individual decision as to whether or not that physician, institution, or hospital shall associate professionally with chiropractors. Individual choice by a medical physician voluntarily to associate professionally with chiropractors should be governed only by restrictions under state law, if any, and by the individual medical physician's personal judgment as to what is in the best interest of a patient or patients. Professional association includes referrals, consultations, group practice in partnerships, Health Maintenance Organizations, Preferred Provider Organizations, and other alternative health care delivery systems; the provision of treatment privileges and diagnostic services (including radiological and other laboratory facilities) in or through hospital facilities; association and cooperation in educational programs for students in chiropractic colleges; and cooperation in research, health care seminars, and continuing education programs.

An injunction is necessary to assure that the AMA does not interfere with the right of a physician, hospital, or other institution to make an individual decision on the question of professional association.

Form of Injunction

1. *The AMA, its officers, agents and employees, and all persons who act in active concert with any of them and who receive actual notice of this order are hereby permanently enjoined from restricting, regulating or impeding, or aiding and abetting others from restricting, regulating or impeding, the freedom of any AMA member or any institution or hospital to make an individual decision as to whether or not that AMA member, institution, or hospital shall professionally associate with chiropractors, chiropractic students, or chiropractic institutions.*

2. *This Permanent Injunction does not and shall not be construed to restrict or otherwise interfere with the AMA's right to take positions on any issue, including chiropractic, and to express or publicize those positions, either alone or in conjunction with others. Nor does this Permanent Injunction restrict or otherwise interfere with the AMA's right to petition or testify before any public body on any legislative or regulatory measure or to join or cooperate with any other entity in so petitioning or testifying. The AMA's membership in a recognized accrediting association or society shall not constitute a violation of this Permanent Injunction.*

3. *The AMA is directed to send a copy of this order to each AMA member and employee, first class mail, postage prepaid, within thirty days of the entry of this order. In the alternative, the AMA shall provide the Clerk of the Court with mailing labels so that the Court may send this order to AMA members and employees.*

4. *The AMA shall cause the publication of this order in JAMA and the indexing of the order under "Chiropractic" so that persons desiring to find the order in the future will be able to do so.*

5. *The AMA shall prepare a statement of the AMA's present position on chiropractic for inclusion in the current reports and opinions of the Judicial Council with an appropriate heading that refers to professional association between medical physicians and chiropractors, and indexed in the same manner that*

*other reports and opinions are indexed. The court imposes no
restrictions on the AMA's statement but only requires that it
be consistent with the AMA's statement of its present position
to the court.*

6. *The AMA shall file a report with the court evidencing compliance with this order on or before January 10, 1988.*

It is so ordered.
Susan Getzendanner
United States District Judge
September 27, 1987[1]

9

THE RAINBOW

The AMA was between a rock and a hard place. If they settled, they would be accused of being soft. If they filed an appeal, it was likely that they would continue to get beaten up in court. At this point, they were defeated, and I think they knew it. But the AMA decided to fight to the end.

They appealed Judge Getzendanner's verdict, but we felt confident that the Court of Appeals would let it stand. Judge Getzendanner had made a solid case and I felt sure that the Court of Appeals would affirm her decision. Just under three years later, on February 7, 1990, the United States Court of Appeals for the Seventh Circuit did just that: It upheld the federal district court ruling that held the AMA *et al.* guilty of violating the Sherman Antitrust Act by engaging in an illegal boycott of the chiropractic profession. This, for us, represented the most critical victory of our lawsuit.

While the district courts decide individual cases, based on facts and legal procedure, decisions by Courts of Appeals set precedents upon which other cases are judged—in effect, their affirmation of a decision makes it law. This law becomes binding on all the district courts within an appeals court's circuit, and becomes very persuasive in all the other circuits as well. The Court of Appeals found that the conspiracy against chiropractic did indeed constitute an antitrust injury, rather than a free speech issue, as the AMA claimed. From an antitrust perspective, one of the best portions of the opinion from the appellate court read as follows [all emphasis added]:

Relief here is provided not only to the plaintiff chiropractors, *but also in a sense to all consumers of health-care services.* Ensuring that medical physicians and hospitals are free to professionally associate with chiropractors (e.g., by the publication and mailing of the order to AMA members) likely will eliminate such anticompetitive effects of the boycott as interfering with *consumers' free choice in choosing a product (health-care provider) of their liking.* In this way competition is served by the injunction. In short, the injunction, as designed by Judge Getzendanner, reasonably attempts to eliminate the consequences of the AMA's boycott, and we will not disturb it.[1]

The immediate result of the Court of Appeals' decision was that the AMA was forced to abide by the terms of Judge Getzendanner's injunction (see page 173). Now the American Medical Association had two options. They could file a motion asking all eleven Court of Appeals judges to hear the pleading for a retrial. Or they could ask the United States Supreme Court to stay the injunction and ultimately hear the case. With either choice, their chances of reversing the ruling were slim.

The AMA chose the second option, the appeal to the United States Supreme Court. In November 1990, the Supreme Court declined to hear the case, in effect deciding to let Judge Getzendanner's ruling stand and affirming the verdict of the Court of Appeals. At last, the result was final: *We had won!*

* * *

There was still work remaining to be done between George McAndrews, on behalf of the plaintiffs, and the legal representatives for the defendants. There was no question that the American Medical Association would have to pay. We had waived any claim for punitive damages, but the AMA was still liable for our litagation costs. The question now to be resolved was: How much? A monetary figure had to be thrashed out and a settlement agreed upon by both parties.

Some of the most active work was spent on this phase of the case, and it drove our legal costs up considerably. At the same time, members of the chiropractic profession, having heard that the lawsuit had been won, stopped contributing money to the National Chiropractic Antitrust Committee. Voluntary contributions came to an abrupt halt. Yet it would have been unwise to take action to urge the profession to keep the money coming; if we did, we would alert the defendants to the fact that we were faced with an economic crunch, and this might encourage them to be that much more disagreeable and difficult in reaching a settlement. The game-playing did not end with the verdict.

Finally, after very intense negotiations, the AMA agreed to a monetary settlement, but as part of the agreement insisted that the cash amount must not be disclosed. The settlement was to be disbursed through George McAndrews to the National Chiropractic Antitrust Committee in installments over a five-year period. Such a stipulation on the AMA's part was understandable. Being forced to pay compensation to the chiropractic victors in the case had to be an embarrassment to them. The organization would not want its members to know how much of their dues was being spent to pay for a battle that had been lost—and, even worse, was going for chiropractic education or research, when the AMA had done such an outstanding job of beating up on chiropractic for so long. With a lump-sum payment, it would have been impossible to hide the bottom line in annual financial reports. With an extended payment schedule, the amount would be somewhat more difficult to track.

The money from the settlement went first to pay legal fees that had not been covered by the voluntary contributions to the National Chiropractic Antitrust Committee. Finally, we were able to reimburse George for his expenses. By this time, the total amount of hourly fees and out-of-pocket expenses that had been accumulating was approaching $1 million. George had agreed not to hold us, the plaintiffs, or the National Chiropractic Antitrust Committee responsible for these charges if donations and/or settlements did not come in to cover them—not because he was so wealthy that he could afford it (he couldn't), but because he had taken the case largely in memory of his late father and on behalf of his father's unjustly maligned profession. If we had not won, this would have put him, his family, and his practice at great financial risk. Except for our attorneys, no individual involved with the suit received, or will ever receive, one penny of the settlement.

Beyond that, the lawsuit had been supported by contributions from the profession, so it was only right that any part of the award not needed to cover legal costs should go back into it. We plaintiffs all agreed to turn the settlement money over to the

NCAC. Once the NCAC had paid all the costs of litigation, the organization's charter provided for the options of either dividing the remaining money equally among all the existing accredited chiropractic colleges, or giving the funds to a tax-exempt organization to be used for chiropractic research.

Having lost the lawsuit, the AMA sought to downplay the defeat and to portray the matter as no big deal. But believe me, it was indeed a big deal. Although no one knows the exact dollar figure for how much the lawsuit cost the defendants, I believe it probably was in excess of $15 million—and I would not be surprised if even this estimate is too conservative, and the real figure is well over $20 million. The costs for our side were a mere fraction of that figure. Just imagine if all the money and energy spent by both sides had instead been put toward research and education, and if instead of seeking to destroy chiropractic, the AMA had simply adopted a policy of acting in the best interest of patients, cooperating and consulting professionally in every way. What an impact that redirection of resources could have had on reducing pain and suffering in this country!

* * *

With victory in the antitrust lawsuit behind us, it might have been expected to be a time of great rejoicing in our camp. And we did rejoice, to be sure, but pleased though we were, for me it became a time to reflect on the past, and how what had happened could be applied to the future. It has been said that as America goes, so goes the world. With respect to health care, the effect our court victory would have upon the future would now become more important than ever before.

The public ignorance and prejudice toward chiropractic that for years had been fed and watered by the AMA were not going to evaporate simply because a federal district court had ruled that the illegal boycott must stop immediately. It takes more than the stroke of a pen to turn off prejudice or eradicate ignorance. Significant damage had been done, and even assertive damage control on our part could not undo it. In all probability, much of the damage would never be corrected; when attitudes are formed in the minds of the people, those attitudes often become too deep-seated to be changed.

The court had recognized this, and had done what was legally possible to address the problem. In theory, the AMA's boycott of chiropractic had ended in 1980, with Report UU (see page 89), but, as the judge noted, there was no explicit statement there that it was indeed ethical for M.D.s to associate professionally with chiropractors. The court, in appraising the evidence—and this was a principal reason that injunctive relief was considered necessary—dismissed the argument that Report UU represented a genuine change of heart on the part of the AMA, saying:

> [Report UU] was obviously written by lawyers in an effort to bring the AMA into compliance with antitrust laws, and not a bold change of position designed to reverse the attitudes of AMA members formed . . . by the then eleven-year-old boycott.[2]

Further, the court concluded that the effects of the boycott persisted because "the AMA has never acknowledged the lawlessness of its past conduct," and noted:

> [T]he AMA had never affirmatively stated that it was ethical for medical physicians to professionally associate with chiropractors; that the AMA had never publicly stated to its members the admissions made in the trial court about chiropractic's improved nature; . . . a medical physician had to read very carefully the current AMA Judicial Council opinions to realize that there had been a change in the treatment of chiropractors.[3]

Without clear proof that the AMA had abandoned its unlawful practices—or, if it had, that it hadn't abandoned them only in anticipation of legal action—the court had to acknowledge the probability that the illegal activities would be resumed.

We had won the lawsuit, but total victory for our cause would come only when the lingering effects of the lengthy boycott were completely eliminated. Incredibly, even after it lost the suit, the AMA still managed to put out negative propaganda about chiropractic, although it was more discreet. For example, it came out with a publication called *Reader's Guide to Alternative Health Methods*, with the subtitle "An analysis of more than 1,000 reports on unproven, disproven, controversial, fraudulent, quack, and/or otherwise questionable approaches to solving health problems."[4] Despite the fact that chiropractic is a bona fide licensed profession and scientifically recognized healing art, this publication contained a section on chiropractic.

Chiropractic's reputation is also hurt, at times, by sensationalist media coverage. Public opinion on many subjects is strongly influenced by information in the media, and on television in particular; unfortunately, with the popularity of talk shows and magazine-type shows, it has become quite lucrative to broadcast material that purports to expose some questionable conduct somewhere in the country, especially if the material is sensational. This is not so much a matter of malice, but rather a function of the way the media operate. The press and the electronic media are greatly concerned with improving circulation and ratings; this enables them to charge higher advertising rates and thus maximize profits. The problem is that objectivity and honesty may be compromised in the process.

For example, *20/20*, a very popular network television program that features a certain style of investigative reporting, aired a segment on chiropractic.[5] When the American Chiropractic Association heard that this program was to be produced, the organization offered its input, but *20/20* declined the offer and chose as its main authority on chiropractic Dr. Murray S. Katz, a Canadian physician who has long been openly and aggressively hostile in his opposition to chiropractic. The same Dr. Katz had previously been questioned under oath for three days and discredited by the government commission that produced the *Chiropractic in New Zealand Report*; he had falsified his credentials to that body, misrepresenting himself as a chiropractor and as the author of a Canadian government report on chiropractic.[6] Katz's vehemence in denouncing chiropractic on *20/20* may have made for good television, but it also created an unbalanced presentation in which facts were lost and obscured, and there was no opportunity for a credible rebuttal on the part of chiropractors. This did a major disservice to viewers, who tend to trust—in this case mistakenly—that journalists have done their homework.

Similarly, the magazine *Consumer Reports* has published reports on treatment for back pain that painted a very negative picture of chiropractic.[7] Not surprisingly, they too relied heavily on the the perspective of M.D.s biased against chiropractic, and neglected to mention the numerous studies that testify to chiropractic's safety and effectiveness. This is particularly unfortunate given the reliance that many Americans place on this publication, believing it to be fair and trustworthy in conducting its various studies.

In short, our profession still has the job of educating and redirecting the thinking in the minds of many people as to what really constitutes rational, safe, and effective health care. We won in the legal arena; now we need to win in the public arena.

10

A NEW DAY
IN HEALTH CARE

W hen we filed the lawsuit against the American Medical
Association and the other defendants on Columbus
Day, October 12, 1976, we had little idea what would
ultimately be in store for us. But perhaps the bliss of ignorance
actually helped us to move forward without hesitation. We had
estimated that the suit would take, at most, two to five years to
resolve. How wrong we were, and how slowly justice moves!

Still, it was well worth it, to say the least. The result was a
blistering defeat for the American Medical Association, a vindi-
cation of the chiropractic profession, and—most important of
all—a victory for freedom of choice in health care. In the final
analysis, what matters is not so much the conduct of the AMA
or how a handful of chiropractors triumphed over that organization in court, nor even the courage of a brilliant attorney who
was willing to put everything he had on the line for an honorable
cause. What is most important is the need of the American
people for an approach to health care that objectively assesses
and then utilizes the best treatments available, regardless of
what they may be. This means cooperation among practitioners
of all state-licensed health care professions. The success of our
lawsuit finally opened the door to the possibility of constructive
professional relationships between chiropractors and other
health care professionals.

With over 57,000 members worldwide, chiropractic is the
largest drug-free health care profession in the world. It sub-
scribes to a wellness- and prevention-oriented approach that
stresses the importance of body structure as it affects body

function and health. A chiropractor does not treat ailments as such. Rather, he or she treats *the patient for the ailment,* with emphasis on the role of the spine and nervous system.

The following is a list of some of the ailments for which patients consult chiropractors most frequently:

- Lumbago.
- Headache.
- Limb pain.
- Backache (unspecified).
- Neck sprains and strains.
- Neck pain.
- Lumbar sprains and strains.
- Muscle pain (unspecified).
- Lumbosacral sprains and strains.
- Lumbar vertebral disorders (multiple and ill-defined locations).[1]

Chiropractic treatment is designed to enhance a patient's inherent recuperative ability. The human body has a natural tendency toward homeostasis—that is, to maintain a uniform and beneficial physiological stability. Chiropractic adjustment is intended to assist the body in this ability.

Like orthodox medicine, chiropractic does not have all the answers to every health problem, but where it does, it is without equal.

* * *

Experts in the field of communication teach that for an idea to be accepted by society, it must be reinforced by "multiple channels of communication"—for example, radio, TV, newspapers, billboards, junk mail, word of mouth, and so on—plus pervasiveness, repetition, and a high profile. According to Philip Lesly, author of *Lesly's Handbook on Public Relations and Communication,* once these things are achieved, the idea will "pass through the veil of resistance and cynicism and will be adopted by the people."[2] This formula does not consider the truth of the idea, only how an idea must be marketed so that it is accepted.

The marketing of ideas effectively programs how we think. We tend to think of programming as something that affects only the weak, or people trapped in religious cults, or possibly those subjected to deliberate brainwashing of some type. But in fact it affects us all to some extent, no matter how intelligent we are.

During World War II, the Nazi government included a Minister of Propaganda by the name of Joseph Goebbels. He was extremely talented as a propagandist, and all news media throughout the Third Reich had to clear their reports and information through his office. Thus, he was able not only to conceal from the German public some of the horrendous things being perpetrated by Hitler's government, but also to exaggerate reports of victories, so that the German people sincerely believed they were winning the war long after the tide had turned for them.

I once read that near the end of the war, a ship set sail for the United States with a group of German prisoners of war on board. These were no ordinary prisoners, but members of the high command of the Third Reich. They were being brought to the United States for interrogation. Near the end of their voyage, they were given a fine meal, and they began sneering at the Americans for giving them this food. The Americans could not understand why their generosity was regarded with such contempt. The Germans then said that they knew the Americans did not have an abundance of food sufficient to give them such a meal, and that obviously the Americans must be patronizing them because the roles of captor and captive would soon be reversed. The Americans insisted they were wrong, but the Germans wouldn't hear of it. Finally, an American officer said, "All right, you can see for yourself, when we pull into New York Harbor tomorrow."

"Never!" they cried. "You will never pull into New York Harbor. We have seen pictures of your city in ruins, and you will never let us see this destruction!" It turned out that in Berlin, they had been shown photographs of what were supposed to be the bombed ruins of New York City. The Germans openly laughed at the Americans, who insisted that the city had never been bombed.

As promised, the ship approached New York City the next day, and as it pulled into the harbor, the Germans looked at the city with wonder and disbelief. One of the Americans, satisfied that the Germans must finally recognize that they had been victims of misinformation, asked, "Well, what do you think of your Dr. Goebbels now?"

Puzzled by the question, the Germans looked at the American, and one of them asked, "We don't understand. What does Dr. Goebbels have to do with this?"

The American officer replied, in exasperation, "Then why are you all staring at the skyline with such disbelief and amazement?"

Another of the Germans answered, "American ingenuity, that they could rebuild this city so quickly!"

The Germans were so well programmed that they couldn't see a truth as large as New York City. Were they stupid? Not at all. They were intelligent people, but they had been so completely programmed that their brains refused to recognize the truth, even though it should have been painfully obvious to them.

In the case of health care, we are forever being sold on the idea that taking care of ourselves means using the tools of modern medicine, particularly drugs. Got a cold? Just take one of these cold pills and the symptoms will go away for awhile. Headache? There are all kinds of pills for that. Indigestion? Don't worry about eating that extra slice of pizza—one of these pills will make you feel better. Can't sleep at night? Just take one of these sleeping pills. Aches and pains? No problem, we've got pills for that, too. The advertisements for these products are not likely to mention that good nutrition, rest, exercise, and other common-sense measures may be just as effective. It's not in the interest of the advertisers. And while the various companies advertising these products would, no doubt, say they are merely informing the public about the benefits of individual products, the underlying message—especially when you consider the volume of drug advertising we all encounter—is that when something ails you, the appropriate response is to take some type of medication for it. Ultimately, medical doctors are the beneficiaries of this as well, since they are the ones who write the prescriptions.

For certain types of disorders, drugs can be life-saving. The problem is, however, that we have been taught to see drugs as the best treatment for *all* health problems. In the case of a problem involving chronic pain, such as back pain or headaches, this can be particularly dangerous. It is not uncommon to see people start on a course of relatively mild painkillers and then gradually move up to stronger and stronger ones, as the pills become less effective, until eventually dependency or even physical addiction results. I am forever grateful that I was saved from traveling down this road by Walter Kopec, the pharmacist who asked me to think about whether I really wanted to take the painkiller my doctor had prescribed. If he had not done so, chances are I might never have discovered chiropractic, which not only relieved my back pain (without side effects or the danger of addiction), but also became my life's work.

Many, if not most, Americans have not been so fortunate. The American people have undergone heavy programming in their attitudes toward health care. Programming can block out all logic and common sense, and programmed people recognize only what the programmer wants them to see. Thus many people believe orthodox medical care is the only choice they have. A person who is suffering from pain may go to a doctor, who will examine her and authorize all sorts of invasive, uncomfortable, and expensive tests, then tell her, "I can't find anything wrong with you. You're getting older, you know, and these things are normal." Even though the patient knows that what she is feeling is *not* normal, she will nod and accept the diagnosis and her own discomfort for a period of time—a year, or maybe two, until her chronic condition rears its head in some other way, such as in persistent headaches, an inability to sleep, or some other intolerable symptom. And then she will try again, probably with another doctor. If she tries long and hard enough, she might eventually opt for a type of treatment outside the scope of orthodox medicine. But relatively few people do, because nothing and no one within the medical establishment helps them to arrive at this point.

This is a lingering effect of the AMA's attempt to destroy the practice of chiropractic in the United States. For decades, unnoticed and unhindered, the orthodox medical establishment has limited our right to choose among the various approaches to health care. This has created a public that for the most part knows only how to be good medical patients. Faced with different modalities of treatment, we choose medicine not necessarily because it is the best care, or even a logical choice, but because we have been programmed to think of health care as consisting of drugs and surgery. This programming has been so pervasive and successful that people who advocate other approaches to health care are often met with sneers and disbelief—like those of the German prisoners as they approached New York Harbor. Sadly, many people stubbornly close the door on superior methods of health care that do not fit the traditional mold, and as a result deprive themselves of the best possible treatments for their particular ailments.

Although we won a major battle on behalf of chiropractic, we must nevertheless continue to fight the war—the war against ignorance and prejudice in health care. Ignorance and prejudice often die hard, but with education and cooperation, minds can be opened. Licensed health care providers of all disciplines must put past differences behind them and join hands to serve suffering humanity. Ideally, members of all healing professions should learn about each other's practices, and understand the advantages of all possible approaches. This would bring honesty and objectivity to health care, and benefit not only individual patients, but the health care system as a whole.

* * *

Health care and health care reform have been much-debated topics in recent years. Many people feel that when it comes to health care, they are paying more and more and getting less and less. There is evidence that they are right. If grocery prices had gone up at the same rate as health care costs over the past sixty years, we would now be paying $14.83 for a roll of toilet paper, $36.67 for a pound of coffee, $45.83 for a dozen eggs, $58.33 for a pound of butter, and $61.66 for a dozen oranges.[3]

One key aspect of the reform we need in health care is both very simple and extremely difficult; it is a real paradox. The simple part is the concept that all health care providers must use honesty, objectivity, common sense, and compassion in dealing with their patients. The difficult part is the change of heart that is required if physicians are to abandon the pursuit of protectionism and focus instead on seeing that their patients receive the best and most appropriate care.

One of the major factors behind today's health care cost woes is that there has been a sort of professional monopoly among doctors. As with all monopolies, this stifles competition, and when there is no competition, prices rise and quality suffers. My experience over many years of professional practice, and the many things I learned in the course of the lawsuit against the AMA, have led me to the conviction that if this situation is to be changed, there must be reform in four general areas:

1. *Reform in the minds of the general public.* The public needs to realize that there are choices to be made in health care, and that these choices should be made on the basis of what has been shown to be effective. With regard to one of the available choices, chiropractic care, the public must learn that it has been proved to be a safe and effective form of health care for neuromusculoskeletal ailments, and that the reason many people do not take it seriously is nothing more or less than an extremely well organized and financed plan to discredit and destroy the chiropractic profession that was orchestrated by the American Medical Association and its allies. The United States Federal Court affirmed this fact by finding the AMA guilty of violating the Sherman Act.

2. *Reform in the minds of the government.* This requires an honest and courageous effort on the part of legislators to speak out openly for the intelligent utilization of all licensed forms of health care treatment based on their merits, not preexisting bias. Many political leaders in the United States, as well as members of their families, have personally utilized chiropractic care and recognize its value. Many have even come to chiropractic conferences and conventions as guest speakers, and spoken glowingly about the effectiveness of chiropractic. Unfortunately, all too often, these same prominent figures fail to use their positions of influence to say the same to the public at large. This is all the more ironic as we keep hearing of the general "health care crisis" and the ever-looming bankruptcy of Medicare and Medicaid. Chiropractic has been shown to be not only safer and more effective than conventional medical care for certain health problems, but far more *cost*-effective.[4] If chiropractic care were routinely used where it is appropriate, an enormous number of health care dollars could be saved and put to better use. For example, people with back pain and other structurally related ailments should be directed to outpatient chiropractic care, rather than toward hospitalization and surgery. Eight out of ten people

have a low back problem at some time in their lives, and the average total cost for a typical lumbar disc operation comes to approximately $60,000, so you don't need a degree in economics to see the enormous savings this could yield.[5] It should be emphasized that this is not an issue of chiropractic *versus* medicine, but of utilizing all of the various valuable health care modalities at the appropriate times, based on the therapeutic benefits of each.

3. *Reform in the minds of the medical profession.* The medical profession must learn to accept the fact that it does not always have the best answer to every health care problem, and it must learn to embrace and work with other professions that offer different strengths—among them chiropractic, which has been shown to be a superior form of treatment for certain neuromusculoskeletal ailments. Government agencies from around the world, including Great Britain, Canada, and New Zealand—and finally now the U.S. Agency for Health Care Policy and Research (AHCPR)—have found that spinal manipulation is a superior treatment for low back pain.[6] Unfortunately, the response among certain members of the medical community has been anything but accepting. In fact, soon after the AHCPR guidelines came out, that government agency found itself the target of a lobbying group, headed by an orthopedic surgeon, that is working to have the agency's funding discontinued.[7] If we are to have rational health care, and get the best possible care for the greatest possible number of Americans, the medical profession must stop living in the past with respect to chiropractic. Medical physicians must learn that their type of health care is not the only way, but that there are other methods that can be superior for certain problems. Hospitals must open themselves up to include chiropractic within orthopedic departments. We must all embrace an ethic of interprofessional cooperation if we are to deliver better, safer, and more cost-effective health care. As we know, the AMA's record in this regard is hardly exemplary. Either the leaders of the medical profession must change their attitudes or the medical profession must change its leaders.

4. *Reform in the minds of chiropractors.* The chiropractic profes-

sion must take responsibility for proclaiming the truth about chiropractic, and it must hold itself to the highest possible standards at all times. In the past, the profession has tended to respond to criticism by first apologizing and then quietly recommitting itself to professional excellence, hoping that public approval and acceptance by the medical leadership would follow. A commitment to professional excellence is certainly noble and honorable, and I feel it has become a hallmark of the chiropractic profession. But the willingness of chiropractors to tolerate the many lies printed and told about it has always been an enigma to me. I compare this situation to that of a small country with a large, hostile neighbor that bombs the smaller nation's cities and then condemns and ridicules it for having rubble its streets—except that some chiropractors would even apologize for the rubble! Of course, no profession is without its shady characters and eccentrics, and it is for these individuals that we often feel a need to apologize. But the way to deal with that problem is to have the professional leadership take a firm stand against the individuals who are at fault—not to feel that there is something wrong with the profession as a whole. Dishonesty and eccentricity are not chiropractic problems (or for that matter, medical problems); they are *human* problems. However, because of the legacy of misinformation and propaganda that continues to shadow chiropractic, we must be particularly concerned to isolate suspect practitioners from the profession lest they take the entire chiropractic profession down with them.

Low back pain is one of the most expensive health care problems in America today. It costs some $20 billion a year for medical care, plus an additional $50 to $60 billion a year in lost productivity.[8] It is the second most common ailment that sends patients to primary health care providers.[9] Low back disc surgery is the third most common type of surgery done in the United States, after tubal ligation and cesarean section.[10]

Between 250,000 and 350,000 disc surgeries were performed in 1993.[11] Yet according to a report on the *CBS This Morning*, as many as 80,000 of these surgeries were *unnecessary*.[12] Most chiropractors would probably say that this figure is way too low, and that more than half of the people who have undergone disc surgery could have been helped by the more conservative (and less dangerous and expensive) outpatient care provided by chiropractors.

There are numerous studies that support this:

• Studies of workers' compensation records from the states of California and Oregon showed that chiropractic offers a 2-to-1 superiority—both therapeutically and economically—over conventional medical care for low back pain.[13] A similar study of the records of the Utah State Workers' Compensation Board found a 10-to-1 economic advantage for chiropractic care of low back pain. Time lost from work cost an average of $68.38 for patients receiving chiropractic care and $668.39 for patients receiving medical care.[14]

• The *Chiropractic in New Zealand Report 1979* concluded, among other things, that chiropractic was "an impressively safe and clinically effective form of health care," and insisted that medical and chiropractic doctors must work together.[15]

• AV-MED, the largest health maintenance organization (HMO) in the southeastern United States, referred 100 patients with low back pain to the Silverman Chiropractic Center in Miami for treatment. Prior to receiving chiropractic treatment, all but 20 of the patients had been treated by an M.D.; 2 had been hospitalized and 12 had been diagnosed as needing disc surgery. After chiropractic treatment, *none* required surgery. The HMO estimated that utilizing chiropractic treatment had saved hundreds of thousands of dollars and, more important, saved many people from having to endure unnecessary hospitalization and surgery.[16]

• Per Freitag, M.D., observed orthopedic patients in two Chicago hospitals, one of which used chiropractic care, and concluded that chiropractic care could shorten the average hospital stay by seven to nine days.[17]

• An Italian study found that chiropractic care reduced the number of hospitalizations by 87.6 percent and the average amount of time lost from work by 75.5 percent.[18]

• A study reported in the *Western Journal of Medicine* in 1989 found that chiropractic patients were three times more satisfied with their care, on average, than were patients of family practice physicians.[19]

• A ten-year government-sponsored randomized controlled trial study conducted by a British medical doctor, T.R. Meade, found that for patients with chronic low back pain, chiropractic outperformed medical care by as much as a 2-to-1 margin.[20] A follow-up study of all of the 741 patients three years later showed that the outpatient care in chiropractic offices was 29 percent more effective than hospital medical care at providing continuing relief of pain.[21]

• The Canadian government commissioned a study led by a noted economist, Pran Manga, Ph.D., of the University of Ottawa. After researching all available literature, clinical studies, and statistical and other pertinent data, he concluded that there was "an overwhelming body of evidence indicating that chiropractic management of low-back pain is more cost-effective than medical management."[22]

• In 1991, the world-renowned RAND (Research and Development) corporation released the results of a study that found spinal manipulation to be an "appropriate" treatment for back pain. Indeed, the head of the study, Dr. Paul Shekelle, said in an interview on the ABC television show *20/20,* "There are considerably more randomized controlled trials which show the benefit of [chiropractic] than there are for many, many other things which physicians and neurosurgeons do all the time."[23]

Probably the most impressive endorsement of chiropractic to date comes from the Agency for Health Care Policy and Research, a division of the U.S. Department of Health and Human Services' Public Health Service. In December 1994, this organization issued a series of publications to serve as guidelines for clinicians and patients. The guidelines, entitled *Acute Low Back Problems in Adults,* clearly recommend spinal manipulation as the treatment of choice for most cases of low back pain.[24] They do not mention chiropractic by name, but 94 percent of spinal manipulations are performed by chiropractors.[25] Moreover, since the guidelines state that spinal manipulation "should only be done by a professional with experience in manipulation," the implication is obvious.[26]

The AHCPR guidelines were produced by a panel of twenty-three health care providers and other professionals (twelve of them M.D.s) who conducted a scientific study, including extensive literature searches, of the effectiveness of available treatments for acute low back pain. The panel consulted with an additional 200 experts from around the world who went through tens of thousands of research articles dealing with low back pain. Once the guidelines were developed, they were subjected to peer review and pilot testing to verify their validity. It is worth noting that the AHCPR guidelines not only recommend spinal manipulation as a treatment for back pain, but also discourage the use of disc surgery, even in cases of a herniated (ruptured) disc. In fact, they point out, "Surgery has been found to be helpful in only 1 in 100 cases of low back problems. In some people, surgery can even cause more problems. This is especially true if your only symptom is back pain."[27]

This is an entirely new emphasis on conservative approaches in the treatment of low back pain. It constitutes a radical departure from the past. Of course, physicians are not required to follow these guidelines, but they do carry significant weight. Specifically, a doctor who ignores them may run the risk of inviting malpractice lawsuits for being too hasty with surgery, especially if surgery is unsuccessful or if complications ensue.*

The United States Department of Defense has become interested in chiropractic as well, and is undertaking what it calls its Chiropractic Health Care Demonstration Program. This calls for giving chiropractic treatment to patients in ten military hospitals and comparing their experiences with those of patients in three other military hospitals who do not receive chiropractic treatment. It has been forty years since I worked in the medical department at Fort Lewis, Washington, where I administered what may have been some of the first chiropractic treatments ever given on an army base—always taking great care to get medical authorization, so as

---

*As one might have predicted, many surgeons were quite unhappy about the new guidelines, and interestingly, the AMA produced its own *Pocket Guide to Back Pain* (Random House, 1995) soon after the AHCPR guidelines came out. This publication, which claimed to present "the latest on all treatment options" never mentions spinal manipulation. Meanwhile, a group headed by an orthopedic surgeon began to actively lobby in Washington to destroy the AHCPR, calling it "an unnecessary bureaucracy that publishes inferior clinical practice guidelines" and an "agency that has outlived its usefulness." (*Dynamic Chiropractic*, 25 September 1995.)

not to risk being disciplined for using unorthodox procedures. All I can say is that it has been a long time in coming.

*   *   *

One day, after we had finally won the lawsuit against the American Medical Association, George McAndrews and I were talking about success, and what it meant to each of us. I asked George what his definition of success was. He said, "Simply having no regrets. This doesn't mean not having any failures, but adapting failures into the human experience, and knowing that you have done your best in life."

I liked his definition, and I jotted it down. It started me thinking. Like most people, I guess I had tended to think of success simply as accomplishing a chosen task. Now I was beginning to see it as a progressive realization of worthy goals— goals that are never final, but that continue to evolve as part of an ongoing process for as long as we live. To say that you have "succeeded" or "arrived" would be to put brakes on the wheels of progress. For us, winning the lawsuit was merely another part of the journey in the right direction, not an end in itself. There will always be new challenges and higher goals as we move through life.

I will have accomplished my purpose in writing this book if you find, after reading it, that:

• You have become aware of the fact that you *do* have the right to choose among different forms of health care.

• You have learned of the benefits of chiropractic care for back pain and other structurally related ailments, and have been freed from the grip of medical programming concerning chiropractic.

• You are motivated to write letters to your legislators urging that chiropractic be included in all health plans and tax-exempt hospitals.

• You are prepared to demand that chiropractic care be utilized in all hospitals and covered by all health insurance, as a part of a total health care plan.

To most chiropractors, this profession is far more than a job or a means of making a living—it is a way of life. And there is more and more evidence all the time to confirm what chiropractors have always known. Chiropractic is achieving unprecedented acceptance in the minds of informed people—and in general, the more informed people are, the more accepting they are.

Chiropractic has truly come of age. We are proud of everything it represents—the concept of total health care and health maintenance—and we are proud of the fight we won against the medical monopoly that conspired to destroy our profession.

Appendix I

PARTIAL LIST OF STUDIES ON CHIROPRACTIC

Agency for Health Care Policy and Research, *Acute Low Back Problems in Adults*, U.S. Department of Health and Human Services, Rockville, MD, December 1994. A multidisciplinary panel of twenty-three health care professionals (twelve of them M.D.s) and consumer representatives conducted worldwide literature searches and used critical reviews and syntheses to evaluate the effectiveness of available treatments for acute low back pain. In addition, they had the support of 200 medical experts from around the world to research tens of thousands of pieces of literature from scientific journals. Peer review and pilot testing were subsequently used to evaluate the validity and utility of the panel's conclusions in clinical practice. The AHCPR recommended spinal manipulation, together with the use of over-the-counter analgesics, as the treatment of choice for acute low back pain; simultaneously, the panel discouraged the use of disc surgery, except in cases where serious spinal pathology or nerve root dysfunction is found, and it found that traction, massage, diathermy, ultrasound, cutaneous laser treatment, biofeedback, and transcutaneous electrical stimulation (TENS) have not been proved effective for the treatment of low back pain. Since chiropractors provide 94 percent of all spinal manipulation in the United States, this study places chiropractic at the forefront as the preferred treatment approach.

Boline, Patrick D., D.C., Kassem Kassak, Ph.D., Gert Bronfort, D.C., Craig Nelson, D.C., and Alfred V. Anderson, D.C., M.C., "Spinal Manipulation vs. Amitryptyline for the Treatment of Chronic Tension-type Headaches: A Randomized Clinical

Trial," *Journal of Manipulative and Physiological Therapeutics* Vol. 18 No. 3 (March/April 1995), pp. 148–154. A randomized controlled trial conducted at Northwestern Chiropractic College in Bloomington, Minnesota, compared the effectiveness of spinal manipulation with that of amitriptyline therapy. Subjects were 150 patients between the ages of eighteen and eighty. At the end of the four-week treatment period, both modalities were found to have been effective at reducing pain, amitriptyline slightly more so than manipulation. However, four weeks after the cessation of treatment, the subjects who had received amitriptyline had returned to pre-treatment pain levels, whereas those who had received chiropractic treatment experienced continuing relief. Moreover, the incidence of unpleasant side effects was 82.1 percent in the amitriptyline group versus only 4.3 percent for the spinal manipulation group.

Cassidy, David, D.C., and W.H. Kirkaldy-Willis, M.D., University of Saskatchewan Medical Clinic and Research Center, 1985. In a group of 171 chronically (seven years) disabled, medically unresponsive, low back pain sufferers, significant results were seen within two to three weeks under chiropractic care. The prolonged benefits of this chiropractic care were documented as the patients remained pain-free one year later. Dr. Kirkaldy-Willis is a world-renowned medical orthopedist.

Dabbs, Vaughan, D.C., and William J. Lauretti, D.C., "A Risk Assessment of Cervical Manipulation vs. NSAIDs for the Treatment of Neck Pain," *Journal of Manipulative and Physiological Therapeutics* Vol. 18 No. 8 (October 1995), pp. 530–536. A search of scientific literature concerning the risks of spinal manipulation and of the use of nonsteroidal anti-inflammatory drugs (NSAIDs) for the treatment of neck pain compared the rates of serious complications or death from both treatments. The NSAIDs were found to be associated with a very low risk of serious complications or death. However, cervical manipulation was found to be as much as 400 times *less* likely than NSAID use to result in serious complications.

Davis, Herbert, M.D., AV-MED Health Maintenance Organization, Miami, Florida, 1982. The medical director of the largest health maintenance organization in the southeastern United

States conducted a study of 100 patients referred to a chiropractor, Dr. Mark Silverman. Eighty patients in this group were categorized as "medical failures," and had seen an average of 1.6 M.D.s without results. Twelve patients had been diagnosed as needing disc surgery. *All twelve* of the disc problems were corrected in chiropractic treatments without surgery. None of the 100 patients was made worse. The medical director concluded that chiropractic saved $250,000 in costs for the HMO and avoided its operating at a loss. This figure does not include the savings in pain, suffering, and medical complications.

Ebrall, Phillip, D.C., Director, Australian Center for Chiropractic Research, Royal Melbourne Institute of Technology, *Australian Worker's Compensation Study*, 1991. A study compared an equal number of cases of work-related low back injuries without fractures; 998 chiropractic cases were compared with 998 cases drawn at random from a group of 3,712 medical cases. The study concluded that:

1. The average treatment cost per injury under chiropractic care was $392, while under medical care the average cost was $1,569.

2. Time loss in the chiropractic group was 6.25 days per injury, compared with 25.56 in the medical group.

3. Acute patients (patients with symptoms that are more severe but of shorter duration) receiving chiropractic care had six times less risk of becoming chronic (experiencing symptoms for ninety days or longer).

Freitag, Per, M.D., Ph.D., John F. Kennedy Hospital, Chicago, and Lutheran General Hospital, Park Ridge, Illinois. A professor and leading Chicago-area orthopedic surgeon and radiologist recounted in testimony before U.S. District Court in *Wilk* et al. v. *American Medical Association* et al. his comparision of results in two Chicago area hospital orthopedic wards with patients suffering from low back pain. One of the hospitals used chiropractic care within their ward and other used only medical treatments. His review of patient records concluded that patients receiving chiropractic care were released without pain in five to seven days compared with fourteen days for patients receiving medical care. This demonstrated a 2-to-1 superiority of chiropractic care for patients with low back pain.

The Gallup organization, *Demographic Characteristics of Users of Chiropractic Services,* 1991. A nationwide demographic study compiled by the Gallup organization reported that 90 percent of chiropractic patients surveyed felt the treatments they received were effective; 80 percent of those surveyed stated that chiropractic treatments fulfilled most of their expectations.

Jarvis, Kelly, D.C., Reed Phillips, D.C., and Elliot Morris, J.D., M.B.A., "Cost per Case Comparison of Back Injury Claims of Chiropractic Versus Medical Management for Conditions With Identical Diagnostic Codes," *Journal of Occupational Medicine* Vol. 33 No. 8 (August 1991), pp. 847–852. A study of 3,062 nonsurgical back ailments in the 1986 Utah workers' compensation records showed that chiropractic outperformed medicine by a 10-to-1 margin in compensation costs. Patients receiving medical care averaged twenty-one days lost from work and $668.39 for compensation costs for work time lost; patients receiving chiropractic care averaged less than three days lost from work and $68.38 paid for compensation.

Manga, Pran, Ph.D., Doug Angus, M.A., Costa Papdopoulos, M.H.A., and William Swan, B.A., *The Effectiveness and Cost Effectiveness of Chiropractic Management of Low Back Pain.* University of Ottawa, 1993. Epidemiological and health economics literature, and statistics from worker's compensation boards in Canada and other countries were reviewed. The study concluded that chiropractic was *markedly superior* to medical management for low back pain in terms of safety, effectiveness, cost-efficiency, and patient satisfaction. It urged the government to encourage and prefer chiropractic care over medical care for low back pain and recommended that chiropractors be retained by all hospitals as "gatekeepers" to direct the care of patients with low back problems in hospitals. It concluded that chiropractic care could save the government "hundreds of millions of dollars per year."

Martelletti, P., D. LaTour, and others, "Spectrum of Pathophysiological Disorders in Cervicogenic Headache and Its

Therapeutic Indications," *JNMS* 3(4), 1995. A chiropractic and medical research team treated a group of thirty-six patients with cervicogenic headaches (headache caused by problems affecting the nerves in the neck) with a course of twelve cervical manipulations (one adjustment three times weekly for four weeks). Patients kept daily diaries recording the frequency, duration, and intensity of their headaches, as well as their use of painkillers. Immediately following the initiation of chiropractic treatment, a decline in both pain index and drug consumption was recorded, and these remained significantly lowered both after the four week course of treatment and after four weeks of subsequent follow-up. Consequently, the researchers suggested, "cervicogenic headache should be treated with spinal manipulation before the recommendation of invasive techniques." A neck muscle at the base of the skull has attachments to the highly sensitive brain lining (dura mater), which, if irritated by muscle contraction, becomes a basis for cervicogenic headaches.

Martin, Rolland A., M.D., Medical Director, Workmen's Compensation Board, State of Oregon, *A Study of Time Loss Back Claims*, 1971. A total of 237 back injury claims were studied over a period of one year. The average age of claimants was 40 years, and the ratio of male to female claimants was 8 to 1. The majority of patients received various conservative forms of therapy, but of interest to the board were the results of those treated by chiropractic physicians. Eighty-two percent of those workers resumed work after one week of time loss without a disability award. The study also determined that "examining claims treated by an M.D., in which the diagnosis seems comparable to the type of injury suffered by the workmen treated by the chiropractor, forty-one percent of these workmen resumed work after one week of time loss."

Meade, T.W., FRCP. British Medical Research Council, 1990. A government study of 741 patients in eleven hospitals and chiropractic clinics throughout Britain, conducted over a ten-year period, used randomized controlled trials and the scientifically accepted Oswestry Scale for pain measurement to compare chiropractic to physiotherapy. Results were evaluated by Ph.D.s who acted as independent referees. The study concluded that chiropractic care was more effective than medical care for back pain by as much as a 2-to-1 margin. The results of the study made national headlines in England.

A follow-up study of the 741 patients three years later showed that the outpatient care in chiropractic offices was 29 percent more effective than hospital medical care at providing continuing relief of pain.

RAND, Santa Monica, California, 1992. The internationally known and respected nonprofit research group conducted an exhaustive study of scientific literature using a panel of experts including neurologists, medical orthopedists, and chiropractors. They concluded that spinal manipulation, as done by chiropractors, is an appropriate treatment for low back disorders. Paul G. Shekelle, M.D., M.P.H., a principal participant in the study, said, "There are considerably more randomized controlled trials which show the benefit of [chiropractic adjustments] than there are for many, many other things which physicians and neurosurgeons do all the time."

Royal Commission of Inquiry on Chiropractic in New Zealand, *Chiropractic in New Zealand Report 1979.* The government of New Zealand appointed a commission to study chiropractic. The investigative team of this extensive, twenty-month study cross-examined hundreds of leading educators, doctors, and researchers from Australia, Canada, the United Kingdom, and the United States to compile 3,638 pages of transcripts. The commission concluded that chiropractic is a "vital, effective, impressively safe, scientifically based profession." It further recommended that, in the interest of patients, chiropractic be included in all hospitals. The results of this study prompted the British government to conduct its own study on chiropractic (See Meade, T.W., above).

Splendori, F., *Chiropractic Therapeutic Effectiveness—Social Importance, Incidence on Absence from Work and Hospitalization,* Milan, Italy, 1988. An unpublished government-sponsored survey of 17,142 patients over a two-year period showed that chiropractic care reduced hospitalization by 87.6 percent and work loss by 75.5 percent. The study involved chiropractors in twenty-two medical back pain clinics and was done in cooperation with leading universities, which provided scholars with Ph.D.s to be used as independent referees and to record the results over the course of the study.

Wolf, C. Richard, M.D., with special credit to Dr. Floyd R. Hill, *Industrial Back Injury,* California workmen's compensation study of cases in 1972, using information from the Division of Labor Statistics, State of California, 1975. This study compared time loss for cases of back injury (as reported by patients) for individuals treated by medical doctors with those treated by chiropractors. One thousand employees with industrial back injuries reported to the California Division of Labor Statistics were questioned about the time lost and residual pain from their injuries. Half of these injuries were reported as having been treated by medical doctors, the other half by chiropractors. Responses were obtained from 629 patients. The the results were as follows:

• Average lost time per employee: 32 days in the M.D.-treated group; 15.6 days in the chiropractor-treated group.

• Employees reporting no lost time: 21 percent in the M.D.-treated group; 6.7 percent in the chiropractor-treated group.

• Employees reporting lost time in excess of sixty days: 13.2 percent in the M.D.-treated group; 6.7 percent in the chiropractor-treated group.

• Employees reporting complete recovery: 34.8 percent in the M.D.-treated group; 51 percent in the chiropractor-treated group.

This study, like the Oregon Workers' Compensation Board study, reported that chiropractic care may be able to return people to work in half the time and at half the cost of medical care.

Appendix II

LIST OF CHIROPRACTIC COLLEGES IN THE UNITED STATES AND CANADA

Chiropractic colleges in the United States are accredited by the Council on Chiropractic Education, which is the accrediting agency approved by the U.S. Department of Education. The following chiropractic colleges have achieved accreditation:

Cleveland Chiropractic College
6401 Rockhill Road
Kansas City, MO 64131

Cleveland Chiropractic College
590 North Vermont Avenue
Los Angeles, CA 90004

Life Chiropractic College
1269 Barclay Circle
Marietta, GA 30060

Life Chiropractic College–West
2005 Via Barrett
P.O. Box 367
San Lorenzo, CA 94580

Logan College of Chiropractic
1851 Schoettler Road
P.O. Box 1065
Chesterfield, MO 63006

Los Angeles College of Chiropractic
16200 East Amber Valley Drive
Whittier, CA 90604

National College of Chiropractic
200 East Roosevelt Road
Lombard, IL 60148

New York College of Chiropractic
P.O. Box 800
Seneca Falls, NY 13148-0800

Northwestern College of Chiropractic
2501 West 84th Street
Bloomington, MN 55431

Palmer College of Chiropractic
1000 Brady Street
Davenport, IA 52803

Palmer College of Chiropractic–West
1095 Dunford Way
Sunnyvale, CA 94087

Parker College of Chiropractic
2500 Walnut Hill Lane
Dallas, TX 75229

Sherman College of Straight Chiropractic
2020 Springhill Road
Spartanburg, SC 29304

Texas Chiropractic College
5912 Spencer Highway
Pasadena, TX 77505

University of Bridgeport
College of Chiropractic
75 Linden Avenue
Bridgeport, CT 06601

Western States Chiropractic College
2900 NE 132nd Avenue
Portland, OR 97230

Canadian Memorial Chiropractic College
1900 Bayview Avenue
Toronto, Ontario M4G3E6

Appendix III

NATIONAL CHIROPRACTIC ASSOCIATIONS

During its growth, chiropractic has felt the growing pains typical of all healing professions. As a result, the chiropractic profession today is represented by two national chiropractic associations:

American Chiropractic Association
1701 Clarendon Boulevard
Arlington, VA 22209
(703) 276–8800

International Chiropractors Association
1901 L Street NW, Suite 800
Washington, DC 20036
(202) 659–6476

Although differences of opinion on certain issues have existed (and still do exist) within the profession, there has consistently been agreement on the basic principles of chiropractic.

The American Chiropractic Association (ACA), the larger of the two professional chiropractic organizations, characterizes chiropractic as follows:

Chiropractic is a branch of the healing arts which is concerned with human health and disease processes. Doctors of chiropractic are physicians who consider man as an integrated being, but give special attention to spinal mechanics, musculoskeletal, neurological, vascular, nutritional, and environmental relationships. (*ACA Master Plan*, ratified June 1964, amended June 1979.)

Of the techniques and practice of chiropractic, the ACA says:

The practice and procedures which may be employed by doctors of chiropractic are based on the academic and clinical training received in and through accredited chiropractic colleges. These shall include, but are not limited to, the use of diagnostics and therapeutics. Such procedures specifically include the adjustment and manipulation of the articulations and adjacent tissues of the human body, particularly of the spinal column. Included is the treatment of intersegmental disorders for alleviation of related functional disorders. Patient care is conducted with due regard for environmental, nutritional and psychotherapeutic factors as well as first aid, hygiene, sanitation, rehabilitation, and physiological therapeutic procedures designed to assist in the restoration and maintenance of neurological integrity and homeostatic balance. (*ACA Master Plan,* ratified June 1964, amended June 1977.)

The ACA defines the underlying principle of chiropractic as follows:

Chiropractic is based on the premise that the relationship between structure and function in the human body is a significant health factor and that such relationships between the spinal column and the nervous system are the most significant, since the normal transmission and expression of nerve energy are essential to the restoration and maintenance of health. (*ACA Master Plan,* ratified June 1964, amended June 1975.)

In the same vein, the International Chiropractors Association says:

I. The SCIENCE of chiropractic deals with the relationship between the articulations of the skeleton and the nervous system, and the role of this relationship in the restoration and maintenance of health. Of primary concern to chiropractic are abnormalities of structure or function of the vertebral column known clinically as the vertebral subluxation complex. The subluxation complex includes any alteration of the biomechanical and physiological dynamics of contiguous spinal structures which can cause neuronal disturbances.

II. The PHILOSOPHY of chiropractic holds that the body is a self healing organism and that a major determining factor in the development of states of disease or dysfunction is the body's inability to comprehend its environment either internally and/or externally. Directly or indirectly, all bodily function is controlled by the nervous system, consequently a central theme of chiropractic theories on health is the premise that abnormal bodily function may be caused by interference with nerve transmission and expression due to pressure, strain or tension upon the spinal cord, spinal nerves, or peripheral nerves as a result of a displacement of the spinal segments or other skeletal structures (subluxation).

III. The ART of chiropractic pertains to the skill and judgment required for the detection, location, analysis, control, reduction and correction of primarily the vertebral subluxation complex. It also involves the determination of any contraindications to the provision of chiropractic care or to any particular method.

The ICA holds that the chiropractic spinal adjustment is unique and singular to the chiropractic profession due to its specificity of application and rationale for application. (*International Chiropractors Association Policy Handbook Code of Ethics*, 3rd ed., 1993.)

As is evident from these passages, there is great commonality between the views of the two organizations as to the fundamentals of what chiropractic is and how it works.

NOTES

Throughout these notes, "*Wilk* v. *AMA*" denotes *Wilk* et al. v. *American Medical Association* et al., United States District Court for the Northern District of Illinois, Eastern Division, Civil Action No. 76 C 3777.

Chapter 1
Before the Storm
1. S.I. McMillen, *None of These Diseases* (Old Tappan, NJ: Fleming H. Revell Company, 1968), p. 1315.

   Howard Haggard, *Devils, Drugs and Doctors* (New York: Harper and Brothers, 1929), pp. 85–93.

   Morton Thompson, *The City and the Covenant* (New York: Signet Books, 1969).

Chapter 2
A Cloud of Propaganda
1. William Kitay, *The Challenge of Medicine* (New York: Holt, Rinehart and Winston, 1963), p. 21.
2. Batten and Associates, Inc., *Chiropractic Survey and Statistical Study* (Des Moines, IA: Batten and Associates, 1963), pp. 34–35, 36–37.
3. John McMillan Mennell, M.D., testimony entered as evidence in *Wilk* v. *AMA*, 6–7 May 1987. From transcript of proceedings before District Judge Susan Getzendanner, p. 2089.
4. "Independent Practitioners Under Medicare," Health, Education, and Welfare Secretary's Report to the Congress (Washington, DC: U.S. Department of Health, Education, and Welfare, 28 December 1968).
5. Joseph A. Sabatier, M.D., editorial, *Journal of the American Medical Association* Vol. 209 No. 11 (16 September 1969).
6. "Why Chiropractic Cult Cannot Provide Quality Health Care," *Senior Citizens News* Vol. 2, No. 88 (January 1969), p. 1.
7. Ibid.
8. Ibid., p. 2.
9. Health Insurance Association of America, position statement on coverage of

services of limited practitioners, 19 February 1969.

10. Ralph Lee Smith, *At Your Own Risk: The Case Against Chiropractic* (New York: Pocket Books, 1969), p. 10.

11. Ronnie Joan Mark, Librarian, *Medical World News* (New York, NY), letter to Chester Wilk (Park Ridge, IL), 19 January 1973.

12. Tryon Edwards, *The New Dictionary of Thoughts*, revised and enlarged by C.N. Catrevas, Jonathan Edwards, and Ralph Emerson Browns (StanBook, Incorporated, 1977), p. 60.

13. George Seldes, ed., *The Great Quotations*, 7th ed. (New York: Simon & Schuster, 1972), p. 798.

14. Howard Wolinsky and Tom Brune, *The Serpent on the Staff: The Unhealthy Politics of the American Medical Association* (New York: Jeremy P. Tarcher, Inc., 1994), p. 128.

15. American Medical Association Committee on Quackery, memorandum to the American Medical Association Board of Trustees, 4 January 1971. Quoted in William Trever, *In the Public Interest* (Los Angeles: Scriptures Unlimited, 1972), pp. 4, 29. Also Plaintiff's Exhibit 1338 in *Wilk* v. *AMA*.

16. American Medical Association Committee on Quackery, memorandum to the American Medical Association Board of Trustees, 4 January 1971. Quoted in Trever, *In the Public Interest*, p. 124.

17. American Medical Association House of Delegates, official policy statement on chiropractic, adopted November 1966, in American Medical Association, *Opinions and Reports of the Judicial Council* (Chicago, IL: American Medical Association, 1971), p. 15. Quoted in Trever, *In the Public Interest*, p. 56.

18. Trever, *In the Public Interest*, p. 123.

19. George P. McAndrews, Timothy J. Malloy, Charles W. Shifley, Robert C. Ryan, Audrey Horton, Robert H. Resis, and Paul E. Slater, "Plaintiffs' Summary of Proofs as an Aid to the Court," in *Wilk* v. *AMA*, submitted 25 June 1987, pp. 23–35.

20. Robert A. Youngerman, American Medical Association Committee on Quackery, confidential memorandum to H. Doyl Taylor, Department of Investigation, American Medical Association, 21 September 1967. Quoted in Trever, *In the Public Interest*, p. 52.

21. David W. Powers, Director, Management Services Division, American Medical Association, memorandum to AMA Representatives, ca. November 1969–January 1970, pp. 2–3. Reproduced in Trever, *In the Public Interest*, Chapter Four, Documentation.

22. Trever, *In the Public Interest,* pp. 132–133.
23. Minutes of a meeting of the American Medical Association Committee on Quackery held 12 January 1968 at AMA Headquarters, Chicago, IL. Cited in Trever, *In the Public Interest,* p. 41.

   Minutes of a meeting of the American Medical Association Committee on Quackery held 10 May 1968 at AMA Headquarters, Chicago, IL. Quoted in Trever, *In the Public Interest,* p. 41–42.
24. Trever, *In the Public Interest,* pp. 41–42.
25. Seldes, *The Great Quotations,* p. 652.

Inset: *The Relative Safety of Chiropractic*
1. Andreis Kleynhans, "Complications of and Contraindications to Spinal Manipulative Therapy," in *Modern Developments in the Principles and Practice of Chiropractic,* ed. Scott Haldeman (New York: Appleton Century Crofts, 1980), p. 360.
2. Pran Manga, Doug Angus, Costa Papdopoulos, and William Swan, *The Effectiveness and Cost Effectiveness of Chiropractic Management of Low-Back Pain* (Ottawa, Canada: University of Ottawa, 1993).

   T.W. Meade, S. Dyer, et al., "Low Back Pain of Mechanical Origin: Randomised Comparison of Chiropractic and Hospital Outpa-

tient Treatment," *British Medical Journal* Vol. 300 No. 6737 (2 June 1990), pp. 1431–1437.
3. Paul Jaskoviak, "Complications Arising from Manipulation of the Cervical Spine," *Journal of Manipulative and Physiological Therapeutics* 3 (1980), pp. 213–219.
4. David Chapman-Smith, *The Chiropractic Report,* promotional issue (1986).
5. Vaughan Dabbs, D.C., and William J. Lauretti, D.C., "A Risk Assessment of Cervical Manipulation vs. NSAIDs for the Treatment of Neck Pain," *Journal of Manipulative and Physiological Therapeutics* Vol. 18 No. 1 (October 1995), p. 534.

Inset: *How Scientific Is Chiropractic?*
1. William Trever, *In the Public Interest* (Los Angeles: Scriptures Unlimited, 1972), p. 142.
2. Minutes of a meeting of the American Medical Association Committee on Quackery held 6 January 1967 at the Drake Hotel, Chicago, IL, p. 5. Quoted in William Trever, *In the Public Interest* (Los Angeles: Scriptures Unlimited, 1972), p. 13.
3. Segment with guest Paul G. Shekelle, M.D., M.P.H., *20/20,* American Broadcasting Corporation, 4 February 1994.
4. Richard Smith, "Where is the Wisdom. . . ? The Poverty of

Medical Evidence," *British Medical Journal* 303 (6806) (5 October 1991): pp. 798–799.

5. Ibid.

6. David Eddy and J. Billings, *The Quality of Medical Evidence and Medical Practice.* (Washington: National Leadership Commission on Health Care, 1987).

7. Smith, "Where is the Wisdom. . . ? The Poverty of Medical Evidence."

8. Herbert H. Davis, M.D., Medical Director, AV-MED Health Plan (Miami), letter to Mark Silverman, D.C., Silverman Chiropractic Center (Miami), 9 March 1983.

   P.G. Shekelle, A.H. Adams, et al., *The Appropriateness of Spinal Manipulation for Low Back Pain* (Santa Monica, CA: RAND, 1992).

   L.G. Schifrin, *Mandated Health Insurance Coverage for Chiropractic Treatment: An Economic Assessment, with Implications for the Commonwealth of Virginia* (Williamsburg, VA: The College of William and Mary; and Richmond, VA: Medical College of Virginia, 1992).

   D.H. Dean and R.M. Schmidt, *A Comparison of the Costs of Chiropractic versus Alternative Medical Practitioners* (Richmond, VA: University of Richmond, 1992).

Chapter 3
Gathering Thunder

1. "Constitution of the National Chiropractic Antitrust Committee" (Chicago, IL: National Chiropractic Antitrust Committee, 17 October 1974).

2. F. Donnell Hart, Chairman, Congress of Chiropractic State Associations (Holyoke, MA), letter to Chester Wilk (Chicago, IL), 11 October 1975.

3. "Report of the Attorneys for the Congress of State Presidents," read at the closing meeting of the Congress of Chiropractic State Associations, Rosemont, IL, 26 October 1975.

4. Chester A. Wilk, D.C. (Chicago, IL), letter to Harry Rosenfield, Legal Counsel, American Chiropractic Association (Washington, DC), 25 November 1975.

5. Paul Slater, Professor, Northwestern University School of Law (Chicago), personal communication, December 1975.

Chapter 4
The Clouds Roll In

1. American Medical Association Committee on Quackery, memorandum to the American Medical Association Board of Trustees, 4 January 1971. Also Plaintiff's Exhibit 1338 in *Wilk v. AMA.*

2. Ibid.

3. Robert B. Throckmorton, legal counsel, Iowa State Medical Society, "What Medicine Should Do About the Chiropractic Menace," outline of remarks to the North Central Medical Conference spon-

sored by the Iowa State Medical Society, Minneapolis, Minnesota, 11 November 1962. Also Plaintiff's Exhibit 172 in *Wilk* v. *AMA*.

4. Ibid.

5. Notes taken at the *Michigan State Medical Society Chiropractic Workshop*, 10 May 1973 (Lansing, Michigan: Michigan State Medical Society, 1973), p. 2. Also Plaintiff's Exhibit 1288 in *Wilk* v. *AMA*.

6. Michigan State Medical Society, resolution adopted 15 May 1973. Also Plaintiff's Exhibit 1291 in *Wilk* v. *AMA*.

7. American Medical Association House of Delegates, official policy statement on chiropractic, adopted November 1966, in American Medical Association, *Opinions and Reports of the Judicial Council* (Chicago, IL: American Medical Association, 1971), p. 15.

8. American Medical Association, *Principles of Medical Ethics*, (Chicago, IL: American Medical Association, 1957), Principle 3.

9. National Education Association, "Consumer Education," resolution adopted 30–31 March/1 April 1964. Quoted in William Trever, *In the Public Interest* (Los Angeles: Scriptures Unlimited, 1972), pp. 5–6.

10. Samuel R. Sherman, M.D., member, Health Insurance Benefits Advisory Council, U.S. Department of Health, Education, and Welfare (San Francisco, CA), letter to H. Doyl Taylor, Director, Department of Investigation, American Medical Association (Chicago, IL), 11 March 1968. Also Plaintiff's Exhibit 1414 in *Wilk* v. *AMA*.

11. William M. Lees, M.D., "Snap, Crackle, and Pop!" *Illinois Medical Journal* 480.2 (April 1971), pp. 326–332.

12. Health Insurance Association of America, position statement on coverage of services of limited practitioners, 19 February 1969. Also Plaintiff's Exhibits 609 and 616 in *Wilk* v. *AMA*.

13. William R. Hutton, Executive Director, National Council of Senior Citizens, Inc. (Washington, DC), letter to H. Doyle [sic] Taylor, Director, American Medical Association [sic] (Chicago, IL), 2 January 1969.

14. Chester A. Wilk, D.C., deposition in *Wilk* v. *AMA*, 21 February 1978, pp. 181–182.

15. Ibid., pp. 182–184.

16. Ibid., pp. 247–248.

17. Chester A. Wilk, D.C., deposition in *Wilk* v. *AMA*, 19 September 1980, pp. 7–9.

18. Ibid., p. 20.

19. Ibid, pp. 79–80.

20. William M. Lees, M.D., deposition in *Wilk* v. *AMA*.

21. William M. Lees, M.D., "Snap, Crackle, and Pop!" *Illinois Medical Journal* 480.2 (April 1971), pp. 326–332.

22. Wilk, deposition in *Wilk* v. *AMA*, 21 February 1978, pp. 562–570.

23. Settlement agreement exe-
    cuted by George P. McAn-
    drews on behalf of Chester
    A. Wilk, D.C., James W. Bry-
    den, D.C., Patricia B. Arthur,
    D.C., and Michael D. Pedigo,
    D.C., and by the American
    Osteopathic Association, in
    Wilk v. *AMA*, 9 October 1980.

**Inset: *The AMA Reverses Itself
. . . Or Does It?***

1. Board of Trustees of the
   American Medical Association, "Report UU: The Position of the AMA on Chiropractic," adopted by the
   AMA House of Delegates,
   July 1979. Also Plaintiff's Exhibit 7248 in *Wilk* v. *AMA*.

2. Howard Wolinsky and Tom
   Brune, *The Serpent on the
   Staff: The Unhealthy Politics of
   the American Medical Associa-
   tion* (New York: Jeremy P.
   Tarcher, Inc., 1994), p. 138.

3. Betty Jane Anderson, letter to
   John W. Barton, M.D., 26
   May 1981. Also Plaintiff's Ex-
   hibit 7243 in *Wilk* v. *AMA*.

   William B. Smith, letter to
   A.D. Tilgner, 3 May 1985.
   Also Plaintiff's Exhibit 7234
   in *Wilk* v. *AMA*.

   William J. Tabor, letter to
   Kim La Rock, 10 March 1983.
   Also Plaintiff's Exhibit 7245
   in *Wilk* v. *AMA*.

   William J. Tabor, letter to
   Paul F. Tomlin, M.D., 5 May
   1983. Also Plaintiff's Exhibit
   7246 in *Wilk* v. *AMA*.

   Lynn M. Thomas, letter to
   Charles F. Downing, M.D.,
   10 January 1984. Also Plain-

tiff's Exhibit 7220 in *Wilk* v.
AMA.

Chapter 5
The Tempest

1. Michigan State Medical Society, notes taken at the *Michigan State Medical Society Chiropractic Workshop*, 10 May
   1973 (Lansing, Michigan:
   Michigan State Medical Society, 1973), p. 2. Also Plaintiff's Exhibit 1288 in *Wilk* v.
   AMA.

2. Michigan State Medical Society, resolution adopted 15
   May 1973. Also Plaintiff's Exhibit 1291 in *Wilk* v. *AMA*.

3. William M. Lees, M.D.,
   Chairman, Board of Trus-
   tees, Illinois State Medical
   Society (Chicago, IL), letter
   to the University of Illinois
   College of Medicine (Chi-
   cago, IL), 11 June 1974. Also
   Plaintiff's Exhibit 1626 in
   Wilk v. *AMA*.

4. John G. Thomsen, M.D.,
   Chairman, American Medical Association Committee
   on Quackery (Chicago, IL),
   form letter to affiliated medical societies, 1966. Also
   Plaintiff's Exhibits 550 and
   550A in *Wilk* v. *AMA*.

5. Ibid.

6. "AMA Letter Denies Asso-
   ciation Between Physician,
   Chiropractor," *American
   Medical News*, 2 May 1966.
   Also Plaintiff's Exhibit 1467
   in *Wilk* v. *AMA*.

7. J.C. Block, M.D. (Sedalia,
   MO), letter to J.W. Bryden,
   D.C. (Sedalia, MO), 16 No-

vember 1973. Also Plaintiff's Exhibit 174 in *Wilk* v. AMA.

George P. McAndrews, Timothy J. Malloy, Charles W. Shifley, Robert C. Ryan, Audrey Horton, Robert H. Resis, and Paul E. Slater, "Plaintiffs' Summary of Proofs as an Aid to the Court," in *Wilk* v. *AMA*, submitted 25 June 1987.

8. Brian Rovira, M.D., letter to Christopher L. Harrison, D.C. (Tahoe City, CA), 23 January 1974. Also Plaintiff's Exhibits 880 and 798 in *Wilk* v. *AMA*.

9. Otto Arndal, Director, Hospital Accreditation Program, Joint Commission on Accreditation of Hospitals (Washington, DC), letter to Herman D. Meyer, Administrator, Hillcrest General Hospital (Silver City, NM), 9 January 1973. Also Plaintiff's Exhibit 10A in *Wilk* v. *AMA*.

10. Robert B. Throckmorton, Attorney, Judicial Council, American Medical Association (Chicago, IL), letter to members of the American Medical Association, 30 July 1968. Also Plaintiff's Exhibit 253 in *Wilk* v. AMA.

11. Robert B. Throckmorton, legal counsel, Iowa State Medical Society, "What Medicine Should Do About the Chiropractic Menace," outline of remarks to the North Central Medical Conference sponsored by the Iowa State Medical Society, Minneapolis, Minnesota, 11 November 1962. Also Plaintiff's Exhibit 172 in *Wilk* v. *AMA*.

12. Ibid.

13. Ibid.

14. Ibid.

15. Ibid.

16. Henry I. Fineberg, M.D., Executive Vice President, Medical Society of the State of New York (MSSNY), letter to the *Newsletter of the Medical Society of the State of New York*, July 1972. Also Plaintiff's Exhibit 532 in *Wilk* v. *AMA*.

17. David B. Stevens, report concerning announcement in Morehead State University's catalogue of a prechiropractic program, 1969. Also Plaintiff's Exhibit 456 in *Wilk* v. *AMA*.

Harold W. Brunn, letter to William J. Monaghan, 7 August 1972. Also Plaintiff's Exhibit 1519A in *Wilk* v. *AMA*.

18. Royal Commission of Inquiry on Chiropractic in New Zealand, *Chiropractic in New Zealand Report 1979* (Wellington, New Zealand: The Government Printer, 1979).

19. Ibid., p. 106.

20. Ibid., p. 2.

21. Ibid., p. 3.

22. Minutes of a meeting of the American Medical Association Committee on Quackery held at AMA Headquarters, Chicago, IL (no date given). Also Plaintiff's Exhibit 322 in *Wilk* v. *AMA*.

23. Irvin Hendryson, M.D., Member, Board of Trustees,

American Medical Associa-
tion, letter to Robert B.
Throckmorton, General
Counsel, American Medical
Association (Chicago, IL),
1966. Also Plaintiff's Exhibit
241 in *Wilk v. AMA*.

24. Eppie Lederer, *Chicago Sun-Times* (Chicago, IL), letter to
Ernest B. Howard, American
Medical Association (Chi-
cago, IL), 12 August 1974.
Also Plaintiff's Exhibit
1407A in *Wilk v. AMA*.

25. E.S. Crelin, "A Scientific Test
of the Chiropractic Theory,"
American Scientist 61 (1973):
574–580.

26. E.S. Crelin, Professor of Anat-
omy, Yale University (New
Haven, CT), letter to Ray
Sullivan, Executive Director,
Connecticut Medical Soci-
ety, 24 January 1972. Also
Plaintiff's Exhibit 1483A in
Wilk v. AMA.

27. Agreement executed by
George P. McAndrews on
behalf of Chester A. Wilk,
D.C., James W. Bryden, D.C.,
Patricia B. Arthur, D.C., and
Michael D. Pedigo, D.C., and
by the Chicago Medical Soci-
ety, in *Wilk v. AMA*.

Chapter 6
The Eye of the Storm

1. Chester A. Wilk, D.C., testi-
mony in *Wilk v. AMA*, 14
January 1981. From tran-
script of proceedings before
District Judge Nicholas J.
Bua, pp. 4380–4381.

2. Ibid.

3. Robert A. Youngerman, Sec-

retary, American Medical
Association Committee on
Quackery (Chicago, IL),
form letter to affiliated state
medical societies, 1965.

Chapter 7
Quiet After the Storm

1. *American Journal of Public
Health* Vol. 69 No. 5 (1979), p.
439.

2. Martin L. Gross, *The Doctors*
(New York: Random House,
1966), p. 238.

3. William Boyd, *A Textbook of
Pathology: An Introduction to
Medicine* (Philadelphia: Lea
and Febiger, 1961).

4. Ibid.

5. Ibid.

6. E.M. Schimmell, "The Hazards of Hospitalization," *Annals of Internal Medicine*,
January 1964, pp. 100–110.

7. Ibid.

8. Schimmell, "The Hazards of
Hospitalization." Cited in
Martin L. Gross, *The Doctors*
(New York: Random House,
1966), pp. 237–238.

9. Dan Rather, "Is Your Hospi-
tal Safe?" *48 Hours*, CBS
Television Network, 14
September 1995. Cited in
Dynamic Chiropractic, 18
December 1995, p. 2.

10. Howard Hiatt, *The Harvard
Medical Practice Study* (Cambridge, MA: Harvard Uni-
versity, 1990).

11. Public Citizen Congress
Watch, *Medical Malpractice
and National Health Care Reform* (Washington, DC: Public Citizen, July 1993).

12. Public Citizen Congress Watch, *Medical Malpractice and National Health Care Reform.*
    The World Almanac and Book of Facts 1993 (New York: Pharos Books, 1992), p. 698.
13. Luther M. Swygert and Robert A. Sprecher, Circuit Judges, and James E. Doyle, District Judge, decision in *Wilk* v. *AMA*, United States Court of Appeals for the Seventh Circuit, Appeal No. 81-1331, 719 F.2d. 207 (7th Cir. 1983).
14. Settlement agreement executed by George P. McAndrews on behalf of Chester A. Wilk, D.C., James W. Bryden, D.C., Patricia B. Arthur, D.C., and Michael D. Pedigo, D.C., and by the Illinois State Medical Society, in *Wilk* v. *AMA*, 4 March 1985.
15. Ibid.
16. Howard Wolinsky and Tom Brune, *The Serpent on the Staff: The Unhealthy Politics of the American Medical Association* New York: Jeremy P. Tarcher, Inc., 1994), p. 138.

Chapter 8
A Refreshing Rain
 1. John McMillan Mennell, M.D., testimony entered as evidence in *Wilk* v. *AMA*, 6–7 May 1987. From transcript of proceedings before District Judge Susan Getzendanner, pp. 2090–2093.
 2. Per Freitag, M.D., Ph.D., testimony in *Wilk* v. *AMA*, 20 May 1987. From transcript of proceedings before District Judge Susan Getzendanner, pp. 798–885.
 3. Rolland A. Martin, M.D., "A Study of Time Loss Back Claims" (Oregon State Workmen's Compensation Board, March 1971).
 4. Ibid.
 5. C. Richard Wolf, M.D., with special credit to Dr. Floyd R. Hill, "Industrial Back Injury," (California Workers' Compensation Board, 1975).
 6. Ibid.
 7. H. Doyl Taylor, deposition in *Wilk* v. *AMA*, pp. 15, 34–35.
 8. Irvin Hendryson, M.D., member, Board of Trustees, American Medical Association, letter to Robert B. Throckmorton, General Counsel, American Medical Association (Chicago, IL), 1966. Also Plaintiff's Exhibit 241 in *Wilk* v. *AMA*.
 9. Ibid.
10. Ibid.
11. Susan Getzendanner, District Judge, decision in *Wilk* v. *AMA*, 27 August 1987.
12. Committee on Quackery, American Medical Association, memorandum to the Board of Trustees, American Medical Association, 4 January 1971. Quoted in William Trever, *In the Public Interest* (Los Angeles: Scriptures Unlimited, 1972), p. 29. Also Plaintiff's Exhibit 1338 in *Wilk* v. *AMA*.
13. William J. Lynk, testimony in *Wilk* v. *AMA*, 18 May 1987. From transcript of proceed-

ings before District Judge
Susan Getzendanner, pp.
510–517.

14. Royal Commission of Inquiry
on Chiropractic in New Zealand, *Chiropractic in New Zealand Report 1979* (Wellington,
New Zealand: The Govern-
ment Printer, 1979).

15. *Clinical Orthopedics* Vol. 24
(1962), pp. 34–38.
    Royal Commission of In-
quiry on Chiropractic in
New Zealand, *Chiropractic in
New Zealand Report 1979.*

16. Chester A. Wilk, D.C., testimony in *Wilk* v. *AMA,* 21
May 1987. From transcript of
proceedings before District
Judge Susan Getzendanner,
pp. 1086–1099.

17. Ibid.

18. Ibid., pp. 1013–1014.

19. Ibid., pp. 1086–1099.

20. Settlement agreement executed by George P. McAn-
drews on behalf of Chester A.
Wilk, D.C., James W. Bryden,
D.C., Patricia B. Arthur, D.C.,
and Michael D. Pedigo, D.C.,
and by the American Hospital
Association, in *Wilk* v. *AMA,*
12 June 1987, pp. 4–5.

21. Ibid., p. 4.

22. Getzendanner, decision in
Wilk v. *AMA.*

23. Ibid.

24. Settlement agreement exe-
cuted by George P. McAn-
drews on behalf of Chester
A. Wilk, D.C., James W. Bry-
den, D.C., Patricia B. Arthur,
D.C., and Michael D. Pedigo,
D.C., and by the American
College of Radiologists, in

Wilk v. *AMA,* 24 September
1987, pp. 3–4.

25. Settlement agreement executed by George P. McAn-
drews on behalf of Chester
A. Wilk, D.C., James W. Bryden, D.C., Patricia B. Arthur,
D.C., and Michael D. Pedigo,
D.C., and by the American
College of Surgeons, in *Wilk*
v. *AMA,* 24 September 1987.

26. Ibid.

27. Agreement executed by
George P. McAndrews on
behalf of Chester A. Wilk,
D.C., James W. Bryden, D.C.,
Patricia B. Arthur, D.C., and
Michael D. Pedigo, D.C., and
by the American Academy of
Orthopaedic Surgeons, in
Wilk v. *AMA.*

28. Susan Getzendanner, District
Judge, Order of the Court in
Wilk v. *AMA,* 26 September
1987. In compliance with a
court agreement, this document was published in the
*Journal of the American Medi-
cal Association* Vol. 259 No. 1
(January 1, 1988), pp. 81–82;
and in *American Medical
News,* 13 January 1992, pp.
4–5.

29. Ibid.

Inset: *The Boycott of Kentuckiana*

1. Martin Z. Kaplan, M.D. (Lou-
isville, KY), letter to William
J. Monaghan, Department of
Investigation, American
Medical Association (Chi-
cago, IL), 25 January 1969.
Also Plaintiff's Exhibit 251A
in *Wilk* v. *AMA.*

2. Jefferson County Medical Society, resolution addressed to the House of Delegates—Kentucky State Medical Association, on "Kentuckiana Center for Education, Health and Research," adopted 16 February 1978. Also Plaintiff's Exhibit 247 in *Wilk* v. *AMA*.

3. Lorraine Golden, D.C., testimony in *Wilk* v. *AMA*, 1 June 1987. From transcript of proceedings before District Judge Susan Getzendanner, pp. 2143–2150.

Inset: *Text of the Court Order in* Wilk *v.* AMA

1. Susan Getzendanner, District Judge, Order of the Court in *Wilk* v. *AMA*, 26 September 1987.

Chapter 9
The Rainbow

1. Harlington Wood, Jr., Kenneth F. Ripple, and Daniel A. Manion, Circuit Judges, decision in *Wilk* v. *AMA*, United States Court of Appeals for the Seventh Circuit, Appeal Nos. 87-2672 and 87-2777, 7 February 1990.

2. Susan Getzendanner, District Judge, decision in *Wilk* v. *AMA*, 27 August 1987.

3. Ibid.

4. John F. Zwicky, Arthur W. Hafner, Stephen Barrett, and William T. Jarvis, *Reader's Guide to Alternative Health Methods* (Chicago, IL: American Medical Association, 1992), cover.

5. Segment on chiropractic, *20/20*, American Broadcasting Corporation, 4 February 1994.

6. Royal Commission of Inquiry on Chiropractic in New Zealand, *Chiropractic in New Zealand Report 1979* (Wellington, New Zealand: The Government Printer, 1979).

7. "Does Anything Work for Back Pain?" *Consumer Reports*, February 1992.

Chapter 10
A New Day in Health Care

1. American Chiropractic Association Study, quoted in *Journal of American Health Policy*, November/December 1992.

2. Philip Lesly, *Lesly's Handbook on Public Relations and Communication*, 3rd ed. (New York: Amicom Publishing Company, 1983).

3. *Medical Economcs*, 12 September 1994.

4. L.G. Schifrin, *Mandated Health Insurance Coverage for Chiropractic Treatment: An Economic Assessment, with Implications for the Commonwealth of Virginia* (Williamsburg, VA: The College of William and Mary; and Richmond, VA: Medical College of Virginia, 1992).

D.H. Dean and R.M. Schmidt, *A Comparison of the Costs of Chiropractic versus Alternative Medical Practitioners* (Richmond, VA: University of Richmond, 1992).

M. Stano, "A Comparison of Health Care Costs for Chiropractic and Medical Patients," *Journal of Manipulative and Physiological Therapeutics* 16 (1993): pp. 291–299.

5. L. Shvartzman, E. Weingarten, H. Sherry, S. Levin, and A. Persand, "Cost-Effectiveness Analysis of Extended Conservative Therapy Versus Surgical Intervention in the Management of Herniated Lumbar Intervertebral Disk," *Spine* 17 (2) (February 1992), pp. 176–182.

    G.B.J. Anderson, "The Epidemiology of Spinal Disorders," in J.W. Frymoyer, ed., *The Adult Spine: Principles and Practice* (New York: Raven Press, 1991), pp. 107–146.

6. T.W. Meade, S. Dyer, et al., "Low Back Pain of Mechanical Origin: Randomised Comparison of Chiropractic and Hospital Outpatient Treatment," *British Medical Journal* Vol. 300 No. 6737 (2 June 1990), pp. 1431–1437.

    Pran Manga, Doug Angus, Costa Papdopoulos, and William Swan, *The Effectiveness and Cost Effectiveness of Chiropractic Management of Low-Back Pain* (Ottawa, Canada: University of Ottawa, 1993).

    Royal Commission of Inquiry on Chiropractic in New Zealand, *Chiropractic in New Zealand Report 1979* (Wellington, New Zealand: The Government Printer, 1979).

Acute Low Back Problems in Adults: Assessment and Treatment, Highlights from Clinical Practice Guideline Number 14, AHCPR Publication No. 95-0643 (Rockville, MD: Agency for Health Care Policy and Research, Public Health Service, U.S. Department of Health and Human Services, December 1994).

7. "AHCPR Under Seige," *Dynamic Chiropractic* Vol. 13 No. 20 (25 September 1995), p. 44.

8. *Acute Low Back Problems in Adults*, AHCPR Publication No. 95-0642 (Rockville, MD: Agency for Health Care Policy and Research, Public Health Service, U.S. Department of Health and Human Services, December 1994), p. 5.

9. Ibid.

10. Ibid.

11. C.V. Burton and J.D. Cassidy, "Economics, Epidemiology, and Risk Factors," Chapter 1 in W.H. Kirkaldy-Willis and C.V. Burton, eds., *Managing Low Back Pain*, 3d ed. (New York: Churchill Livingstone, 1992), p. 3.

12. Report on unnecessary disc surgery, segment with guest Dr. Robert Poteet, *CBS This Morning*, CBS Television Network, 12 November 1992.

13. C. Richard Wolf, M.D., with special credit to Dr. Floyd R. Hill, "Industrial Back Injury," (California Workers' Compensation Board, 1975).

    Rolland A. Martin, M.D.,

"A Study of Time Loss Back Claims" (Oregon State Workmen's Compensation Board, March 1971).

14. Kelly Jarvis, D.C., Reed Phillips, D.C., and Elliot Morris, J.D., M.B.A., "Cost Per Case Comparison of Back Injury Claims of Chiropractic Versus Medical Management for Conditions With Identical Diagnostic Codes," *Journal of Occupational Medicine* Vol. 33 No. 8 (August 1991), pp. 847–852.

15. Royal Commission of Inquiry on Chiropractic in New Zealand, *Chiropractic in New Zealand Report 1979* (Wellington, New Zealand: The Government Printer, 1979).

16. Herbert H. Davis, M.D., Medical Director, AV-MED Health Plan (Miami), letter to Mark Silverman, D.C., Silverman Chiropractic Center (Miami), 9 March 1983.

17. Per Freitag, M.D., Ph.D., testimony in *Wilk* v. *AMA*, 20 May 1987. From transcript of proceedings before District Judge Susan Getzendanner, pp. 798–885.

18. F. Splendori, "Chiropractic Therapeutic Effectiveness—Social Importance, Incidence on Absence from Work and Hospitalization," unpublished study (Milan, Italy), 1988.

19. D. Cherkin and F. MacCornack, "Patient Evaluations of Low Back Pain Care from Family Physicians and Chiropractors," *Western Journal of Medicine* Vol. 150 (3 November 1989), pp. 351–355.

20. T.W. Meade, S. Dyer, et al., "Low Back Pain of Mechanical Origin: Randomised Comparison of Chiropractic and Hospital Outpatient Treatment," *British Medical Journal* Vol. 300 No. 6737 (2 June 1990), pp. 1431–1437.

21. T.W. Meade, S. Dyer, et al., "Randomised Comparison of Chiropractic and Hospital Outpatient Management for Low-Back Pain from Extended Follow Up," *British Medical Journal* Vol. 311 (1995), pp. 349–351.

22. Pran Manga, Doug Angus, Costa Papdopoulos, and William Swan, *The Effectiveness and Cost Effectiveness of Chiropractic Management of Low-Back Pain* (Ottawa, Canada: University of Ottawa, 1993), p. 13.

23. Segment with guest Paul G. Shekelle, M.D., M.P.H., *20/20*, American Broadcasting Corporation, 4 February 1994.

24. *Acute Low Back Problems in Adults*, Clinical Practice Guideline Number 14.

Acute Low Back Problems in Adults: Assessment and Treatment, Quick Reference Guide for Clinicians.

Understanding Acute Low Back Problems, Consumer Version, Clinical Practice Guideline Number 14, AHCPR Publication No. 95-0644 (Rockville, MD: Agency for Health Care Policy and Research, Public Health Service, U.S. Department of Health and Human Services, December 1994).

25. P.G. Shekelle, A.H. Adams, et al., *The Appropriateness of Spinal Manipulation for Low Back Pain* (Santa Monica, CA: RAND, 1992).

26. *Understanding Acute Low Back Problems,* Consumer Version, Clinical Practice Guideline Number 14.

27. Ibid.

BIBLIOGRAPHY

In addition to the items listed here, sources for this book included the author's personal recollections and communications plus documents, exhibits, files, and court transcripts relating to the case of *Wilk* et al. v. *American Medical Association* et al., United States District Court for the Northern District of Illinois, Eastern Division, Civil Action No. 76 C 3777.

"AHCPR Under Seige." *Dynamic Chiropractic* Vol. 13 No. 20 (25 September 1995): 44.

American Chiropractic Association. *ACA Master Plan.* Arlington, VA: American Chiropractic Association, 1975; 1977; and 1979.

American Medical Association. *Pocket Guide to Back Pain.* New York, NY: Random House, 1995.

Anderson, G.B.J. "The Epidemiology of Spinal Disorders." In *The Adult Spine: Principles and Practice,* ed. J.W. Frymoyer, 107–146. New York, NY: Raven Press, 1991.

Batten and Associates, Inc. *Chiropractic Survey and Statistical Study.* Des Moines, IA: Batten and Associates, 1963.

Boone, Louis E. *Quotable Business.* New York, NY: Random House, 1992.

Boyd, William. *A Textbook of Pathology: An Introduction to Medicine.* Philadelphia, PA: Lea and Febiger, 1961.

Burton, C.V., and J.D. Cassidy. "Economics, Epidemiology, and Risk Factors." In *Managing Low Back Pain,* 3d ed., ed. W.H.

Kirkaldy-Willis and C.V. Burton, Chapter 1. New York, NY: Churchill Livingstone, 1992.

Chapman-Smith, David. *The Chiropractic Report*, promotional issue (1986).

Cherkin, D., and F. MacCornack. "Patient Evaluations of Low Back Pain Care from Family Physicians and Chiropractors." *Western Journal of Medicine* Vol. 150 (3 November 1989): 351–355.

Dabbs, Vaughan, and William J. Lauretti. "A Risk Assessment of Cervical Manipulation vs. NSAIDs for the Treatment of Neck Pain." *Journal of Manipulative and Physiological Therapeutics* Vol. 18 No. 1 (October 1995): 534.

Dean, D.H., and R.M. Schmidt. *A Comparison of the Costs of Chiropractic versus Alternative Medical Practitioners.* Richmond, VA: University of Richmond, 1992.

"Does Anything Work for Back Pain?" *Consumer Reports*, February 1992.

Eddy, David, and J. Billings. *The Quality of Medical Evidence and Medical Practice.* Washington: National Leadership Commission on Health Care, 1987.

Edwards, Tryon. *The New Dictionary of Thoughts.* Revised and enlarged by C.N. Catrevas, Jonathan Edwards, and Ralph Emerson Browns. StanBook, Incorporated, 1977.

Gallup Organization, The. *Demographic Characteristics of Users of Chiropractic Services.* Princeton, NJ: Gallup, 1991.

Gross, Martin L. *The Doctors.* New York, NY: Random House, 1966.

Haggard, Howard. *Devils, Drugs and Doctors.* New York, NY: Harper and Brothers, 1929.

Hiatt, Howard. *The Harvard Medical Practice Study.* Cambridge, MA: Harvard University, 1990.

International Chiropractors Association. *International Chiroprac-*

tors Association Policy Handbook Code of Ethics. 3rd ed. Washington, DC: International Chiropractors Association, 1993.

Jarvis, Kelly, Reed Phillips, and Elliot Morris. "Cost per Case Comparison of Back Injury Claims of Chiropractic Versus Medical Management for Conditions With Identical Diagnostic Codes." *Journal of Occupational Medicine* Vol. 33 No. 8 (August 1991): 847–852.

Jaskoviak, Paul. "Complications Arising from Manipulation of the Cervical Spine." *Journal of Manipulative and Physiological Therapeutics* 3 (1980): 213–219.

Kitay, William. *The Challenge of Medicine.* New York, NY: Holt, Rinehart and Winston, 1963.

Kleynhans, Andreis. "Complications of and Contraindications to Spinal Manipulative Therapy." In *Modern Developments in the Principles and Practice of Chiropractic,* ed. Scott Haldeman. New York, NY: Appleton Century Crofts, 1980.

Lesly, Philip. *Lesly's Handbook on Public Relations and Communication.* 3rd ed. New York: Amicom Publishing Company, 1983.

Manga, Pran, Doug Angus, Costa Papdopoulos, and William Swan. *The Effectiveness and Cost Effectiveness of Chiropractic Management of Low-Back Pain.* Ottawa, Canada: University of Ottawa, 1993.

Martin, Rolland A. "A Study of Time Loss Back Claims." Oregon State Workmen's Compensation Board, March 1971.

McMillen, S.I. *None of These Diseases.* Old Tappan, NJ: Fleming H. Revell Company, 1968.

Meade, T.W., S. Dyer, et al. "Low Back Pain of Mechanical Origin: Randomised Comparison of Chiropractic and Hospital Outpatient Treatment." *British Medical Journal* Vol. 300 No. 6737 (2 June 1990): 1431–1437.

Meade, T.W., S. Dyer, et al. "Randomised Comparison of Chiropractic and Hospital Outpatient Management for Low-Back Pain from Extended Follow Up." *British Medical Journal* Vol. 311 (1995): 349–351.

Public Citizen Congress Watch. *Medical Malpractice and National Health Care Reform.* Washington, DC: Public Citizen, July 1993.

Schifrin, L.G. *Mandated Health Insurance Coverage for Chiropractic Treatment: An Economic Assessment, With Implications for the Commonwealth of Virginia.* Williamsburg, VA: The College of William and Mary; and Richmond, VA: Medical College of Virginia, 1992.

Schimmell, E.M. "The Hazards of Hospitalization." *Annals of Internal Medicine,* January 1964: 100–110.

Shekelle, P.G., A.H. Adams, et al. *The Appropriateness of Spinal Manipulation for Low Back Pain.* Santa Monica, CA: RAND, 1992.

Shvartzman, L., E. Weingarten, H. Sherry, S. Levin, and A. Persand. "Cost-Effectiveness Analysis of Extended Conservative Therapy Versus Surgical Intervention in the Management of Herniated Lumbar Intervertebral Disk." *Spine* 17 (2) (February 1992): 176–182.

Smith, Richard. "Where is the Wisdom. . . ? The Poverty of Medical Evidence." *British Medical Journal* 303 (6806) (5 October 1991): 798–799.

Splendori, F. "Chiropractic Therapeutic Effectiveness—Social Importance, Incidence on Absence from Work and Hospitalization." Unpublished study. Milan, Italy, 1988.

Stano, M. "A Comparison of Health Care Costs for Chiropractic and Medical Patients." *Journal of Manipulative and Physiological Therapeutics* 16 (1993): 291–299.

Thompson, Morton. *The City and the Covenant.* New York, NY: Signet Books, 1969.

Trever, William. *In the Public Interest.* Los Angeles, CA: Scriptures Unlimited, 1972.

U.S. Agency for Health Care Policy and Research. *Acute Low Back*

Problems in Adults. Clinical Practice Guideline Number 14. Rockville, MD: Agency for Health Care Policy and Research, Public Health Service, U.S. Department of Health and Human Services, December 1994. AHCPR Publication No. 95-0642.

Wolf, C. Richard, with special credit to Dr. Floyd R. Hill. "Industrial Back Injury." Sacramento, CA: California Workers' Compensation Board, 1975.

Wolinsky, Howard, and Tom Brune. *The Serpent on the Staff: The Unhealthy Politics of the American Medical Association.* New York, NY: Jeremy P. Tarcher, Inc., 1994.

Zwicky, John F., Arthur W. Hafner, Stephen Barrett, and William T. Jarvis. *Reader's Guide to Alternative Health Methods.* Chicago, IL: American Medical Association, 1992.

INDEX